CORPS
STRENGTH

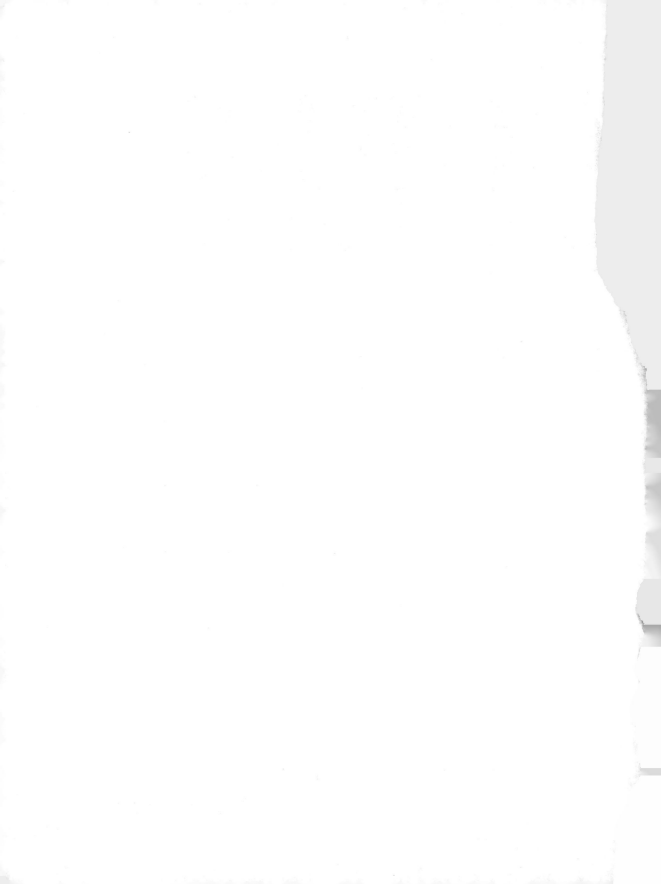

CORPS STRENGTH

A Marine Master Gunnery Sergeant's Program for Elite Fitness

MASTER GUNNERY SERGEANT
PAUL J. ROARKE JR., USMC (RET.)

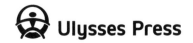 Ulysses Press

This book is dedicated to my parents, Paul and Marcine Roarke.
All I can say is thanks, I love you both very much. PJ

****

Published in the United States by
ULYSSES PRESS
P.O. Box 3440
Berkeley, CA 94703
www.ulyssespress.com

ISBN: 978-1-56975-774-1
Library of Congress Control Number 2009940341

Printed in Canada by Webcom

10 9 8 7 6 5 4 3

Contributing writer: Lori Tubbs ("High-Performance Eating" on page 63)
Acquisitions: Keith Riegert
Editorial/Production: Lily Chou, Claire Chun, Lauren Harrison, Abigail Reser
Index: Sayre Van Young
Design: what!design @ whatweb.com
Photographs: © Rose Spencer except © James Parker on pages 9, 23, 27, 29, 85, 104, 105 and
    back cover; © shutterstock.com/goldenangel (man doing pullup) on front cover; © shutterstock.com/
    Sue Smith, Andresr, Claudio Rossol, Diego Cervo, John Wollwerth, stemack, Fotocrisis, V_Krv, Nick
    Simon, Henrik Winther Andersen, Monkey Business Images on pages 13, 15, 20, 44, 47, 48, 50, 52,
    69, 72, 73; © Paul J. Roarke on pages 61, 75, 76
Models: Paul J. Roarke Jr., Edward Puente, Mario Cummings, Mindaugas Andrelis

Distributed by Publishers Group West

Please Note
This book has been written and published strictly for informational purposes, and in no way should be used as a substitute for actual instruction with qualified professionals. The author and publisher are providing you with information in this work so that you can have the knowledge and can choose, at your own risk, to act on that knowledge. The author and publisher also urge all readers to be aware of their health status and to consult health care professionals before beginning any health program.

TABLE OF CONTENTS

INTRODUCTION:
REAL FITNESS FOR REAL PEOPLE

Before I enlisted in the Marine Corps in 1981, I grew up in a large working-class family in upstate New York. Not many people in this big circle of family and friends went on to college and a white-collar career. The standard career path was a short tour in the military, and then straight to work. They worked with their hands, their heart, and common sense; physical strength, health, and endurance were required to be successful. With skill and honest effort they ran small businesses, worked the fields, and made things of value. Many were construction and factory workers, mechanics, and truck drivers. Some chose to serve as police officers and firefighters. When the call went out, they put aside their tools and served in our military, defending our country against Hitler, communism, and terrorists. It was all work and they did it with humility, integrity, and pride.

Despite the fact that no one really exercised (unless you count hunting and fishing) or followed special diets, you didn't see many overweight people. Nor did you often hear of people being sick. Hurt on the job sometimes, yes, but just at home sick? Almost never. The fact was most of my family never went to the doctor for anything until they were much older, after many decades of hard work. Yet day after day they were able to work hard, raise their families, and stay fairly healthy in the progress. That was the recent past.

In the last 25 years there has been a serious decline in the health and basic fitness of America's working people. It's hard to believe how dramatically the rates of obesity, diabetes, and heart disease have risen over this time period, but don't take my word for it: Go to the Centers for Disease Control's (CDC) website, where they have all the data. It's alarming, but it's all true. Many workers are also getting injured and becoming disabled early in their careers. It's no coincidence that the economic productivity of our country has been waning. Many major American industry icons are also in decline, and in no small part due to the massive increase in the cost of insurance and health care.

The fact is that the health of our nation is directly related to the health and fitness of our people. This is, and has been, the case throughout human history. No great nation has ever survived and prospered when its people were unfit and unhealthy.

Surprisingly, this decline in health and fitness has been accompanied by an explosion of health and fitness products and information. The media is overloaded 24/7 with fitness products, workout DVDs, diet systems, special weight-loss supplements, and more. You'd think that with all this information more available than ever, we'd be in better shape and healthier. The reality, however, is that the opposite is true. While the reasons for this disconnect are pretty simple to explain, it's by no means an easy fix.

Over the past three decades, through much trial and error, I designed a system to get and keep me at a high level of physical fitness for when I couldn't participate in normal Marine Corps training. This is not a standard Marine Corps, body-building or sports-conditioning program. It's a comprehensive system that takes the best parts of many different exercise programs and brings them together to obtain what I call "working fitness." "Working fitness" is a term and goal that I've used for many years. I came up with it to capture the blue-collar nature and goals of the system. Like the working man himself, it's effective, time efficient, and, above all else, results driven.

Throughout this book I'll be running my pie hole, giving my opinions, making observations, and providing recommendations concerning physical fitness and eating—many of which I'm sure that you've never heard before. Or at least never heard explained the way I lay it out. I base 90 percent of my guidance on only three simple things: long personal experience, first-hand observation, and the input of other trusted people. The other 10 percent is what I've read in books (hundreds of them) or heard from what I'd consider a reliable source. Am I hard-headed? Maybe, and while I realize I don't know everything about this subject (far from it), I know what I know. More than anything else, I know what works, and more importantly I know what doesn't work.

I also share many of my experiences related to physical training. "Sea stories" are what we call them in the Marine Corps. Like everything else I write, they have a purpose. Two, actually. One is to illustrate a point I'm trying to make. The second is to entertain you with some funny stuff that I've seen and experienced. I learned a long time ago that when you're instructing or teaching anything, it's best done with real-life examples and humor. Believe it or not, the stories I tell are 100 percent true, to the best of my memory (that's *my* memory).

Another fair warning: I write like I speak, as an adult speaking to other adults. To do it any other way would not be me. So if you don't like direct, honest opinions in "grown folks" language, you need to find another fitness guide.

PART 1
LINE OF
DEPARTURE

CHAPTER 1

WAKE-UP CALL

Of course I didn't know it then, but the first chapter of this book was written when I was around ten years old. It was right about the time my team, the New York Jets, won their only Super Bowl in 1969. For those who weren't there, life for a ten-year-old boy was much different than it is today. First off, there weren't any high-tech toys to keep us indoors. No computers, video games, or iPods. TV—which was essentially cartoons—was limited to a few hours on Saturday mornings. Our parents didn't give much thought to how we spent our free time. They were busy with things like working and keeping the household together. So if the weather was anything short of a hurricane or blizzard, we were pumped full of Cap'n Crunch and booted out the door. We played sports, rode bikes (Sting-Rays mostly), and fished in local ponds. We were like a pack of wild mutts, always moving and looking for something to get into.

The working-class neighborhood where I grew up was filled with kids back then, and there were lots of boys around my age. So a pick-up game of something was never hard to get going. On this particular summer day it was basketball. After throwing fingers to choose sides, we started with a normal driveway game of hoops: lots of missed shots, plenty of fouls, yelling, and attempts at fancy dribbling—not much passing or game plan here. Sounds like fun stuff; however, it seemed like every time I got the ball, one of the other kids just simply grabbed it away from me, or "stuffed it" when I went for a shot.

The bottom line was that I was much smaller than the other kids, shorter by a head, and skinny as a snake. Not that the other kids were young Michael Jordans or anything, but I was damned near a midget compared to them. This happened time and time again, until after one especially nasty blocked shot I reacted like I always did to a physical insult: I took a swing at the kid who did it. Not just some little kid, mind you, but a kid who went on to play college football. He was a few years older, and much bigger than me. Needless to say, in a hot minute I was down, bloodied, with my shirt torn. I somehow managed to tear away, and I ran for home like an escaped mental patient. (If nothing else I could outrun him.) Shouted insults from the boys about my "dwarf" size and "little loser" status followed right behind me.

I reached the house just as my dad was getting home from work, or, as he used to say, "the first shift." My dad owned his own business and routinely worked around the clock. Suppertime was the only chance he had to spend with us. (Work after dinner was the "second shift.") He was unloading some tools from his truck when I ran up, teary eyed, scuffed up, and looking for some sympathy.

Noticing my appearance and bloody shirt, he asked, "What happened to you?"

"I was playing basketball," I blurted. My head was pounding and I could taste blood inside my mouth.

The look on his face told me in a second that he didn't buy that answer. "Huh? I didn't know basketball was such a rough game."

I saw this as my chance, so I unloaded about the game, my lack of size, and my beatdown, leaving out the part about me throwing the first punch. I just wanted some kind of assurance not to worry because I was going to grow up big, and maybe someday even become the best athlete in the neighborhood.

My dad has that personality you'll find in a lot of New York Irishmen. It's a no-nonsense blue-collar way of looking at things, mixed with a smart-ass sense of humor. I noticed he was smiling as he listened and, knowing him, I had a feeling that not much assurance was coming my way. At some point I ran out of breath and stopped ranting. My dad didn't believe in blowing smoke up anybody's rear, and I guess he decided that this was the time I got straightened out on a few things, 10 years old or not.

"Listen, pal," he said with a smile. "You might as well get yourself squared away on this now. You're not built for basketball. You're too short. And you're too small for football. The fact is you're probably going to only be about my size when you grow up."

I had no sense of what that meant, as he was an adult and a giant in my eyes (he was a stocky 5"5' at about 170 pounds).

"Huh? Well, what sport am I built for?" I asked, grabbing for anything positive.

"No sports, my friend. You're really only built for one thing."

"What's that?" I asked anxiously. Jet pilot, frog man, cowboy?

"Years of hard work."

"Hard work? What's that mean?" I asked, dumbfounded.

My dad went on happily. "Hard work. You know, hard physical work." He flexed his big forearm muscle to demonstrate a source of physical labor. He was warmed up now, laughing as he continued. "Like laying bricks, or farm work. Since you're short and built close to the ground, you won't have to bend over very far to pick up stuff. That helps with jobs like moving wheelbarrows full of gravel, or hoeing potatoes. With your build, you'll be able to shovel dirt or split wood all day. You see, being little like you are, it's easy to climb in and around construction sites, in and out of hay barns, up and down ladders, things like that. Short arms are also good for hammering nails and using a paint brush. You'll do fine."

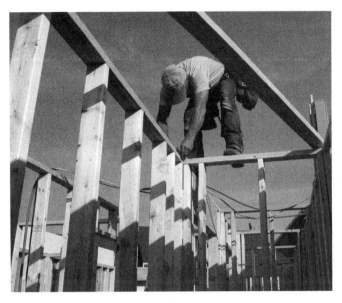

My head was spinning, and I could again feel tears welling up in my eyes (what a great day I was having) as my ten-year-old dreams of playing running back for the Jets or center field with the Yankees were crushed forever. I could now only picture myself as one of the Seven Dwarfs, whistling away as I marched off to work in the mines.

"Oh well," my dad said, sensing my disappointment. "Not everybody has the time to jerk around playing sports. Somebody has to do the work, that's life. It's tough to take sometimes, but it's always going to take effort in any case. If you work hard, you'll always make a living, at least you won't starve. Speaking of that, let's get cleaned up and see what your mother has got for supper."

With that we walked up to the house, ending my first (but not last by a long shot) lesson on the realities of the working man's life. I didn't know till I was much older how much this five-minute conversation would affect me. Looking back, I realize now that this short counseling session (which my dad doesn't even remember) unconsciously set me on a path to prove him wrong, but at the end proved him more right than even he knew at the time.

What is the point of this story? The point is that I want to get something across to you that I learned early in life—that is, not to waste any time trying to cloud an issue, ignore the facts, and make things as you wish they were. First responders, working people, and members of the military depend on their body to make a living, and they need to be and stay in excellent physical condition, whether or not they have to pass an official physical test to be on the job. It's true that all of these different occupations require different levels of fitness. However, in the end they all depend on a body's ability to perform—not just for a short period but for years, really a lifetime. With all that said, you know that you're not going to get in good physical shape or get your weight under control by sitting on your butt whining, making excuses, or wishing it to happen.

I say all this right up front to start helping you get your head right before we spend one second talking about exercising or how to eat right. No pill, rip-off exercise equipment, or secret plant from the Australian outback will do it. I could go on and on with that nonsense. You also have a need that most exercise routines will not prepare you for. The vast majority of exercise and eating programs out there are designed for sports conditioning and/or body building. They aren't the most effective methods for working people. If they were, we wouldn't have so many overweight and out-of-shape people in this country. Need proof? Go to your local mall and just take a good look around. Seeing is believing.

Look, I'm not trying to insult anyone; I just want to get your attention. Losing weight and getting in shape is tough work for anyone, myself included. It always was and always will be hard. This is what I mean by getting your head screwed on right first. If you're in poor physical condition and overweight, you first have to change your thinking. There are no secret exercise routines or some exotic diet that will get you in shape without you putting in the time and effort. Trust me, I know this to be fact not only from my own efforts, but from my observation and training of hundreds of Marines.

As a Marine, I know that an out-of-shape, overweight Marine can put his life and his fellow Marines' lives at risk, and can jeopardize the mission. I also have many friends who are cops and firefighters. They tell me the same thing about the out-of-shape people they work with. I asked one firefighter friend of mine how he could work with firemen who were so out-of-shape and overweight they couldn't be counted on in tough, physically demanding situations. His simple response surprised me.

He said, "Whenever possible, I just make it a point to avoid going into a building with them."

The sad thing is that my law enforcement friends gave me a similar response. If you look at it the right way, people who rely on their bodies to make a living are putting their future, and their families' futures, at risk by not taking care of themselves. It may sound cold but it's all true, and not necessary if people would just get the right (simple) guidance and then make a little honest effort.

Though most people who rely on their bodies for a living realize they need to be in top condition and want to get in shape, they don't have the right guidance, combined with the right mindset, to do so. Military members, first responders, and working people need a physical training system that is designed to provide them with the specific type of conditioning they need. That's why I wrote this book—to cut through the nonsense. I want to make my experience (and the system I developed from it) available to military members, cops, firefighters, construction workers, weekend athletes, and anyone else who wants to obtain a high level of fitness—man or woman, young or old. Here you can learn some simple, tested, and proven methods to get in serious shape, control your weight, *and* become healthier (and happier) along the way.

Another big reason I wrote this book is that I hate to see good people work hard all their lives, doing everything for everyone else. After they've raised their children and done all the right things, they should be ready to enjoy their later years. But most people are physically too worn down, sick, and disabled to do the things they always wanted to do. They (you) deserve better, and with relatively small effort properly applied over the long haul, you can stay strong and healthy for many years. I plan to, and you can, too.

This program makes no distinction between gender, age, physical size, or present fitness levels. It'll work for any healthy person who wants to get in great condition *and* is willing to put in the effort that is required to get there. It can be as tough a program as you want to make it, but not impossible for almost anyone. It just takes some effort, half a brain, and a little faith.

While this program could do great things for almost any healthy person, it won't be for everyone. Many people will feel they don't have the need for a high level of physical fitness, nor will they have the motivation to participate in a program that's not what you'd call exciting nor easy. This program isn't designed to be exciting or easy; its only purpose is to produce results (which is exciting to me): "working fitness" and weight management. Like with anything else worth having, you'll need some self-motivation to make it work.

The intensity level of my exercise routines can be varied from beginners to people already in top condition, and you can easily tailor the sessions to any specific fitness requirement. Combining that with the fact that the sessions are time efficient (you never need more than five hours a week) makes this a universal program for any healthy person. But it's especially effective for military members, first responders, and working people.

It's been my experience that when people fail in their efforts to get in shape and manage their weight, it's not from a lack of effort or even will power. It's usually from a simple lack of knowledge and proper planning. I learned many years ago to "never confuse efforts with results." Results are what count here, and they are the focus of this book. I'll teach you what works and explain why it works. I'll also tell you what doesn't work and why it doesn't work. If results are what you really want, be prepared to work and sometimes be tired, sore, and a little hungry.

All good things in life come with a price tag, so if aren't willing to pay your dues, don't waste your money. You work hard, you get paid; you slack off, you get fired. It's that simple. Basically, the cost of this book is about the same as an order of hot wings and a few beers. If you aren't really going to make an honest effort, forget the book and spend the money on the chow. Hey, I love hot wings and beer, *and* being in shape. Having one doesn't cancel out the other, as you'll learn if you read on. Now hopefully your head is screwed on a little tighter so we can move forward in the right direction. At times we'll stop and adjust along the way, because to take even one step without the right mindset is a step backwards.

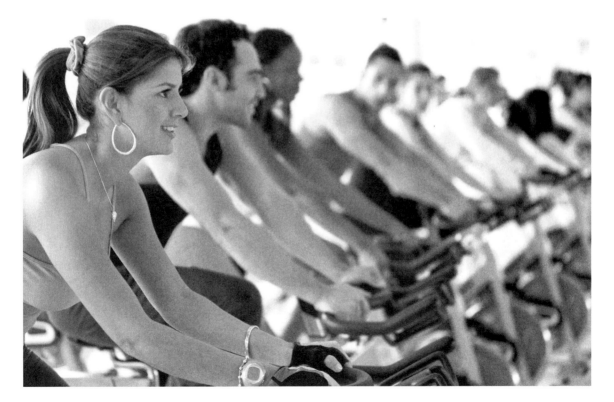

CHAPTER 2

MASTER OF THE OBVIOUS

Like most Marines, during my time in Corps I was given many nicknames. "Rock" was one of my earliest, due to my hard-headedness (and, no, it wasn't because of any low test scores), but there were many others. Trust me when I tell you that most of them were given to bust my chops about something stupid I did or said, not because I did anything special. One that was hung on me years ago was "Master of the Obvious." This was due to my uncanny ability to notice, and then point out, the most obvious things. Rarely did something right under my nose ever escape my notice. It was very funny to many of my friends, and I would laugh as much as any-one when people rode me hard about it, which was basically whenever I did it.

Now, it doesn't sound like much of a superpower to master the obvious, but in reality it's actually quite a useful talent, as it's been my experience that many (most) people miss or misunderstand the most obvious things in life. Physical fitness is no exception, so building on that I'll start with the obvious basics.

All things that last are built on a solid foundation. It doesn't matter what it is: a building, a career, business, a marriage. Same goes for intangible things like ideas and concepts. Anything that you have to rely on must be strongly rooted. The best, strongest foundations are also typically the simplest. The pyramids are over 5,000 years old, but when you get right down to it, they're just large blocks of stone piled on top of each other. However, those blocks were cut with precision from high-quality stone, and then fitted together with great care. That's the difference between a pile of rocks and a pyramid—not easily done by any means, but simple just the same. It's the same for the foundation of health and fitness. I'll break it down for you, as we say in the Marines, "Barney style."

The foundation for health and fitness can only be built on three solid blocks: Half a brain, The RIGHT exercise, and good food.

That's as simple as it gets, and it's *all* you'll ever need. As I said earlier, simple doesn't always mean easy so I'll explain each in detail. I've devoted separate chapters to exercise and eating. The concept of "half a brain" will pop up throughout, so I'll start with that here.

Half a brain? Why not just a brain? Or common sense, education, or basic intelligence? It's because we're talking about getting in shape and getting your weight right, not doing quantum physics or building the space shuttle. You need to put this stuff in its proper perspective. The fact of the matter is, to get into and stay in get great shape needs much less than half your brain. That's a good thing because you need the majority of your brain, your focus, and your energy to manage your life. You have a career, a family, school, bills, etc., to use your brain on. You don't need to waste more than you need on fitness and eating right. You'll need to understand the basics, believe in them, and apply the required effort. They work, long term, and will not need to dominate your life, your thoughts, or all of your spare time.

The longer you do the right things, the sooner they'll become habit and even less of your brain you'll need. For example, remember when you first started driving? You were all keyed up, nervous, and focused only on driving. The road, the other cars, everything—it almost seemed too much to do all at once. Then as time went on and you gained experience, skill, and knowledge about driving, you didn't even think about it (although most people should). You'd think that driving a large, complicated piece of gear like a car down a crowded highway would take 100 percent of your attention. It really doesn't because you know what you're doing, you know how to drive. It's basically the same with working out and eating right. Once you know what you're doing, it'll take minimal attention. But before you get too happy here, remember that it'll take consistent effort, but that in itself is as much a habit as anything else. Being in good shape is as addictive as any drug. The difference is that it takes some initial effort to get the fitness habit embedded, but once it's there, it's there.

To embed the habit of fitness into your life, first understand that working out and eating right need to become part of your life—they're support for your life, NOT your life. This is a very common mistake that'll cause any regime to fail in short order. Your life comes first. I'll say it again and often in this book: YOUR LIFE COMES FIRST. What you need to learn is how to fit exercise and good eating habits around and into your life, not the other way around. Folks like professional athletes, lotto winners, and retired people have the luxury of making working out and eating the focus of their day. You and I don't have that luxury, and you don't need it to get great results.

Here's a good example of what I'm talking about here. Recently, a famous talk show host was all over the media discussing her recent "regain" of about 40 pounds. This is one of the wealthiest women in the world, and her struggles with weight have been well publicized throughout her career. I'm not going to mention her name since I think you know who I'm talking about. Plus, the point isn't to poke fun at her. It's to try and understand her dilemma, as it's common for millions of people across this country.

I recently watched a talk show where her personal trainer, private doctor, and her "spiritual" advisor all talked about her problems with managing her weight. You've got to be kidding me! This person has all that personal support, along with the money to buy the best foods and have it cooked for her by a private chef, and the option to have everything in her life done for her, and she can't get herself in shape? You would think if she can't do it, what chance does an average person—someone who has to work for a living, has limited time and money, and even less energy—have? The simple and obvious answer is that you have an exactly equal chance.

How is that possible? Easy. If you really think about it, all her money, trainers, chefs, doctors, and other advisors won't mean squat (as they don't already) if she can't get her head screwed on right. That's why I stress this more than any other aspect in this book. You have to get your thinking right first, last, and always. You don't have her money, or her high-priced team (why would you want that team?), but hey, you have me. My guidance, combined with the right mindset and some honest effort on your part, is all you really need. (A little patience wouldn't hurt, either.) It'll take you further than any group that she had, for a tiny fraction of what I'm sure she spent. By the way, her trainer sold thousands of books about fitness and nutrition. Would you buy a book from a trainer whose most famous client can't keep herself together with all those advantages? Would you take your car to a mechanic whose own car always stays broken? I wouldn't.

The other reason I use the term "half a brain" is because you don't need to think too much about all this, by which I mean working out and eating right. It's not that complicated, but people tend to overthink things and worry too much about nothing. This "brain overload" causes many to give up before they give it a real chance. You didn't get out of shape overnight, and you're not going to get in shape overnight. The most important thing you need to do is get your thinking right. As far as the rest goes, I've done all the testing and experimenting for you, so save your energy for the effort that's needed, not worry.

CHAPTER 3

PT: PHYSICAL TRAINING

In the Marines we call working out/exercising "PT," which stands for "physical training." For the most part that's how I'll refer to it from here on out, just PT. It's what I know, and to me "working out" sounds more like body building, and "exercising" sounds more like Richard Simmons–type stuff—neither of which are what I'm going to talk about in this book. PT is the right word for my system (which starts on page 26), and I'm all about getting the right mindset first.

Before you embark on any PT/eating plan, it's important to figure out what your goals are first. I mean real goals, not some pie-in-the-sky fantasy. So let me help you out with this, the way I learned it. One night when I was about five years old, the conversation at our dinner table turned to what we (the kids) wanted to do when we grew up. Since I was (am) always anxious to give my opinion, I quickly shouted out, "I want to be an astronaut, or a lumberjack!"

That answer was probably influenced by all the NASA stuff on TV during the 1960s and the recent reading of Paul Bunyan in my kindergarten class. My mom and dad laughed, but then my dad gave me a serious look.

"Well," he said, "You need to figure it out, as there are no trees on the moon, my friend."

In short, get real.

So when you look in the mirror and see that guy or girl looking back at you, realize that it's very unlikely that person is going to be a professional athlete. He or she is probably not going to play pro golf, basketball, football— no, not pro darts—or even professional Monopoly (well, maybe Monopoly). If he or she were, you wouldn't be reading this book, nor would you need to. This book is not for those people. It's for you, me, and all the other working people in the world. So think about your goals in the right way. I'm not saying you shouldn't set a high standard of fitness (or anything else) for yourself. Just use some common sense.

Having said all that, will guidance found in this book make you better at virtually any sport that you choose to play for recreation? Yes, absolutely (on the fitness side, that is; learning the skill part is on you). The methods laid out here can bring you to a very high level of fitness from which you can easily jump off into a more specialized regime for a specific goal, whether it's to run a marathon, race in a triathlon, play touch football, improve your golf game, hike in the mountains, or go cross-country skiing. I've done all those things, and I've also used my own experience playing sports to help me develop this system.

If you're in the military or are a first responder or other hard-working person, we already know that you need to be in shape for your job. Do you also want to lose some weight? Do you play a recreational sport and want to improve your game? Simply speaking, you have to figure out where you want to go before you start moving. It's just like any trip—you pick a destination, plan the route, and get moving in the most direct manner. If you get lost or delayed, stop, figure out the problem, adjust, and get back on track. My system is designed to be flexible in that regard; it can be adjusted for a specific need. Small adjustments will allow almost any healthy person to get maximum benefits from the basic program.

The idea for this system came from where most ideas come from: a need. For me, that need was to maintain a high level of physical fitness for my occupation, which was for almost all of my adult life a United States Marine.

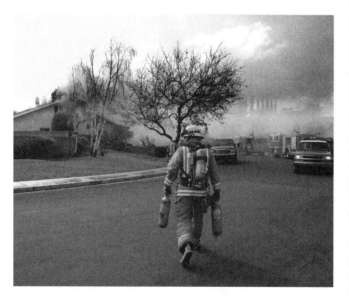

While the Marine Corps has a great physical fitness training program, extensive amounts of traveling and long, irregular hours of working in different places meant I (and many others) had limited time to conduct official PT. Often, we had very little exercise equipment to use. So like any Marine, I improvised, experimented with my own ideas as well as others', observed and noted the results, and made improvements. After many years of trial and error, I came up with this system. I fine-tuned it from my own experiences, but its inherent flexibility leaves it open to be tailored to any individual (or group) needs.

I found that this program also works great for police officers, firefighters, or any job that requires a high level of "working" fitness. It'll improve your overall health and you'll be better able to manage your weight—all of that with the smallest possible investment in time, money, and hassle. You can achieve great results with minimum time because I have cut all the fat, fluff, and wasted time out of this program. It's lean and result oriented, designed to provide a high level of PRACTICAL and USEFUL fitness.

I'm convinced from years of experience that three to five hours a week of the right PT is all you need to stay in great physical condition (assuming you eat like an adult). Keep in mind I'm talking about a high level of fitness here. Not just the ability to walk around the mall or work in the garden, but the real deal. Three to five hours is not a lot of time, not for what you'll get out of it.

Working Fitness

You've heard me use the term "working fitness" several times already, and as you read along you'll find that it's the focus of my program. Before we get into the actual program, you need to understand what I mean by this. Working fitness is really both a concept and a goal. The concept is that it's a type of physical fitness that is first blue-collar in its origin and purpose (meaning it wasn't thought of by some team of MIT professors, exercise doctors, or celebrity trainers, and it's not about professional athletes, movie stars, or models). It's designed for working people, and it all came from one enlisted Marine's head (namely mine) after many years of experience and observation.

I had been doing standard Marine Corps PT for quite a few years when I realized I needed to develop my own training program that would be more effective, flexible, and time efficient. I wasn't really satisfied with the results of the standard program (especially as I got older), and oftentimes we just didn't have time to conduct official PT anyway. In simple terms, what I needed was a program that would "work": work for me, work with my schedule, and get me in the top shape I needed without a lot of special equipment or a big time investment.

That is the concept; the goal was the kind of actual physical ability I was shooting for. For this, I drew on my varied background for the answer. All my life I've played different sports, and I did a lot of construction work before I enlisted in the Marines. After I enlisted, I first served in the Infantry, and later in Aviation Ordnance. These are two very different Military Occupational Specialties (MOS), with very different physical requirements for their actual day-to-day jobs. However, all Marines must pass the same Physical Fitness Test (PFT) and be able to perform basic combat skills regardless of their MOS. As we say in the Corps, "Every Marine a Rifleman." So I wanted to develop a fitness level that would enable me to operate as a Rifleman, an Ordnance man, do well on the PFT, and at the same time do well in any sports I was participating in at the time.

I wanted a 24/7 level of conditioning that would give me the ability to do just about anything, at any given time, and do it all pretty well. I also wanted to have a foundation of fitness that, with a short amount of specialized focus, would allow me to do something specific (like a sport) really well. It had to give me the ability to "work," to get the job done, *whenever* and *whatever* that job may be. Hence the term "working fitness."

To measure working fitness, there are five areas that you need to evaluate:

1. Do you have the ability to effectively perform the actual required tasks of your occupation? Can you really do your job well, and do you feel ready for anything, at any time?

2. Can you demonstrate a high level of performance during any physical testing requirements? All branches of the military and most first responders have annual or semi-annual physical testing evaluations. (By the way, just passing is not a high level of performance to me, and it shouldn't be for you, either. It's a candy-ass move to throw out the age card, or any other excuse, for that matter, as a reason for being overweight or doing poorly on any physical test. You're either in shape or you're not, you're overweight or you're not. You can whine all you want about not being 18 anymore, but the bottom line is there are no "old people," wars, fires, or 911 calls for help. When a firefighter goes into a burning building, a police officer kicks in a door, or a construction worker has to move some equipment, there's no age wavier—you either can do it or you can't.)

3. How well do you perform in any sports or recreational events that you're involved with? Of course, that depends on the sport and how far you want to take it. However, I never met anyone who ran

marathons, triathlons, did martial arts, or played softball/golf/any other sport who didn't want to play well (or win, in other words). As you know, one of the main things of sports is the competition aspect. Yes, it's recreation, but who doesn't want to do well? Anything is more fun when you win.

4. Do you feel good? Are you tired all the time? Do you sleep well? Do you have energy to do the things you want to do? Do you always seem to be sick with something? Listen, hard work makes us all tired—been there all my life. Getting older doesn't make it any easier, either, trust me on that one. We all have aches and pains as we go along, but there is a big difference between being sore and tired from a day of hard work and always feeling exhausted, really injured, and sick all the time. You deserve to feel good and to be able to not just do your job but to enjoy life. So don't ignore the way you feel.

5. With all that, are you maintaining a healthy weight, and is that weight within any standard that you may have to meet for your occupation or for general health?

I used those five measuring sticks to test results of different training efforts over the years. I kept trying different routines and different combinations of ideas till I got to where I wanted to be, or at least pretty close.

It sounds much more complicated than it is. As an example: A six-mile formation run in shorts and sneakers can be a required task in the Marines. So is being able to pass the PFT/CFT and, in my MOS, load heavy ordnance onto aircraft for hours on end. Plus, I had to always keep my weight and personal appearance within standards. These are all required at any given time. But in the end they all require a different type/level of physical fitness, and I wanted to be able to do it all, and not just do it, but do it all really well.

Here are several examples. Can a firefighter in full turn-out gear, with self-contained breathing apparatus, climb ten flights of stairs, break in a door, and then carry an injured person to safety? Does he have the grip strength and endurance to control a high-pressure fire hose for an extended period of time? Can the same firefighter easily pass the Candidate Physical Ability Test (CPAT), which was developed to simulate many different fire-fighting scenarios? Can a police officer defend him/herself against an attack from a violent suspect or pull an injured person from a burning vehicle? Can a welder in a shipyard carry all the heavy gear he needs in and out of tight work spaces, and then move heavy steel plates into position for welding? Can he do this day after day with injuring him/herself, and still have some energy left after a full day to play with his kids?

The point here is that all these people need to develop and know that they have that high level of working fitness before any of those situations comes up. In the end, it's a simple concept. Generally speaking, working fitness must at least include (but is not limited to):

> *"The ability to effectively move your body weight, and to use that body weight to manipulate other items while performing high-intensity short-term and lower-intensity long-term tasks. Working fitness also must include long-term excellent health, weight management, and the capacity to adapt to physical and mental stress."*

In case you're wondering, by themselves athletic ability or body fat content cannot be considered true indicators of working fitness. The other extremely important part of the working fitness concept is that it has to "work" for working people, meaning it can be obtained and maintained without special equipment, lots of time, or even much mental energy (a no-brainer): simple, effective, and time efficient. You'll find that my system is all about working fitness.

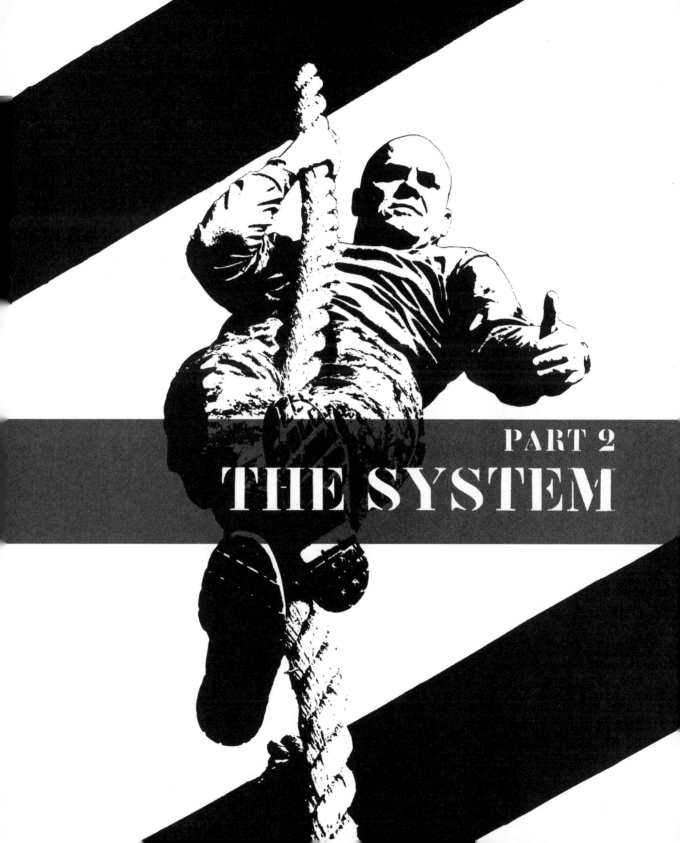

PART 2
THE SYSTEM

OVERVIEW

In the preceding chapters I talked about "working fitness"—what it is and why it's an important goal for people who use their bodies to make a living. So it follows that I designed my system to get you that specific type and level of physical fitness.

I call my method the "Enhanced Physical Readiness System,"™ or EPRS for short. Sounds pretty high speed, huh? Give me a break—I had to call it something, and as a Marine acronyms are what I know, so there you go. But don't worry, the name is about the most complicated part of it. EPRS is divided into three main categories:

A. SAT (Stand Alone Training)

B. Support

C. Active rest

I came up with the terms "SAT," "Support," and "Active rest" to distinguish between the types of physical training (PT) from other methods of exercise you need to get into top shape. All three are important in their own way for health and fitness, and they complement each other when applied the right way.

Before we get into the guts of the system, it's important to put something in perspective. Firefighters, military members, cops, construction workers, etc., are really what I call "working athletes." Professional athletes get paid to perform with their body. If their skill is considerable, they can make a very good living. Some make untold millions, and they all deserve whatever they can get, in my opinion. Their careers are short and often leave them with permanent disabilities. Working people are also athletes in the sense that they must perform with their bodies to earn money, but they don't make millions and their working career is long, really a lifetime. Hence the term "working athlete." I think it's important to keep this in mind as we now go through the actual program. In other words, give yourself some credit, and with that assign some priority to your health and well-being. Not only do you need it, you deserve it.

CHAPTER 4

SAT (STAND ALONE TRAINING)

SAT (Stand Alone Training) is the core of my system and it's pretty simple to get your head around. It needs to be roughly half of the 3–5 hours a week I recommend for PT. SAT is a combination of endurance, strength, and flexibility movements. I call it "Stand Alone Training" because that's what it can do—specifically, give you a high level of working fitness in minimum time, by *itself*. You don't need to do anything else but SAT to get into and stay in great shape. When performed at the right level of intensity with the right balance of time and movements, it'll get you there.

I designed SAT to provide working fitness. Now, there are plenty of other pretty intense physical activities that can get you in pretty good shape, but they lack one or both of the following features, making them less effective than SAT to develop working fitness.

1. They lack balance. In other words, if you just do that activity, you won't get a balance of endurance, strength, and flexibility. For example, I love to ride dirt bikes. For anyone who has done it, riding a large dirt bike over some rough terrain is tough, especially in hot weather. It's a form of exercise, no doubt. But it won't really give you a level of endurance fitness like running. The same goes with running. Running alone is great for aerobic fitness and leg conditioning, but it does very little for upper body strength. The balance of endurance, strength, and flexibility is the first key feature of SAT.

2. They lack flexibility. I've been involved in boxing for over 30 years. It's a great overall body workout. However, it requires specialized gear and some instruction to do it right. So you have to devote a fairly large amount of money to outfit a home boxing gym, or be tied to a boxing gym in both money and the hours that they're open. Either way, you have to get someone to show you how to box. I've been training people to box for years; it's not something you can learn from a book. The same could be said of weightlifting, swimming, martial arts training, yoga, and many other activities, as well as exercise routines like aerobics. They're great overall but have limited flexibility, making them tough to fit into a hectic time schedule. With some very basic knowledge and gear, SAT can really be done almost anywhere, anytime.

The flexibility and balance of this exercise system is derived from its basic make-up. SAT is always made up of the following parts, shown with approximate times. This is based on the one-hour session. (For an explanation of how to break SAT down for shorter sessions, go to Appendix A, page 79.)

1) Warm-up: 5 minutes
2) Pre-Fatigue: 30 minutes
3) Mission: 20 minutes
4) Cool-down: 5 minutes

If done correctly, SAT takes 60 minutes total, and not a minute more.

Now listen closely, sports fans, and get your half a brain working. These times are GUIDELINES; they're what I've developed to make this work within a busy work/life schedule. By sticking closely to these times, you'll also keep your intensity up and get in everything you need. However, don't let these numbers make you mental. If you go over one section by a few minutes, or under in another, it's no biggie, not if you're really pushing yourself. I do it every workout. I doubt if any SAT workout I've ever done has hit each and every timeline exactly; it doesn't need to. However, I do highly recommend that you always use the one-hour maximum as your basic planning tool, especially when you're busy and need to pay close attention to time. At other times when your schedule is more relaxed, you can let your PT run over a little. Not a problem.

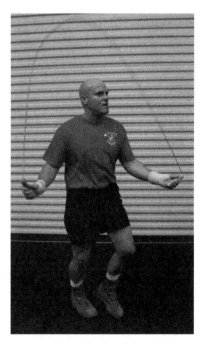

Another reason that I strongly recommend that you try to keep your actual PT to about an hour a session is to prevent overtraining. That's both physical and mental overtraining. I've seen this more times than I can count, and I've made this mistake a few times myself. What happens is people will start out with the best intentions to get into shape and/or lose weight. Many will try to jump right into a very time-consuming and/or complicated routine, normally some advanced routine from a body-building magazine. I'll make a very conservative estimate that 99 times out 100 they never last more than a couple of weeks. The reason is simple: Once you move beyond the effective amount of time required to get into and stay in real shape, you'll become bored and burn out physically and mentally. It's simple human nature. Trust me, you'll find other things to do. The point is to do what is effective for the long term. Working out like a maniac for a couple of weeks, burning out, maybe injuring yourself, and finally giving up is foolish. A hard hour of PT three to five times a week is all you need.

This is the basic outline. Parts 1 and 4 should not change in order or general timelines. Parts 2 and 3 can be done in the laid-out sequence, or combined (I'll explain how) for 50 minutes total. Either way, your goal here is that the total time does not exceed 60 minutes—that's 60 minutes of real work. If you're not completely spent after that hour, you need to raise your intensity level, and I'll give examples of how to do that.

Weighted Vests

All military people and first responders wear heavy protective gear when they go to work. Many other different occupations also require their workers to wear heavy protective gear. Nobody goes into combat/the scene of a fire or accident/crime in progress or works in a steel mill wearing shorts, sneakers, and a tank top. We carry what we need to protect us and to do our job. So you have to train like you fight and work—with your stuff. Or at least with something that simulates that weight. The actual amount of weight, of course, varies with the actual job and/or specific mission.

No matter the weight, there is a right way and a wrong way to train with extra weight. First, you need a high-quality weight vest or a good backpack. A weighted vest designed for this type of training is much better overall. A backpack is good for "humping" (or fast walking/hiking) and maybe doing some short sprints, but it's not designed to be worn while doing exercise movements since it shifts around too much. The best vests are those that allow you to adjust the weight. I've used many brands, but the V-Max is by far the best I've used or seen used. They're made to be worn during PT so that you can do just about any movement without worrying about the weight shifting around. They're high quality and well worth their cost; they'll hold up under hard use and will last many years if you take care of them. I'm not trying to sell you expensive gear, but this is your butt on the line here—get some quality gear so you can train properly. It used to make me mental when I'd hear a Marine complain that some gear/tool we were issued was low quality, but he/she would be wearing a pair of cheap, worn-out running shoes. High-quality training equipment is always a good investment (as long as you use it).

Once you get a weighted vest, you need to wear it periodically during PT to adapt your body to handling the weight. When I say wear it during exercise, I don't mean just putting on a 50-pound weighted vest and running five miles down the road. That'll surely lead to injury, and has been proven many times over. The right way to use a weighted vest is to wear it in a manner that simulates your real-life need, which means for the most part fast walking, short jogs, and stair/hill climbing.

While you could just wear a weighted vest for any standard SAT workout, I think it's more effective to do a specific workout designed for when you wear the vest. Appendix D has three different weighted vest work-

Part 1. Warm-up (5 minutes)

You can find many different opinions about the right way to warm up before exercise. As always, I like to keep things simple and effective so I'll cover some basics about warming up. Warm-ups are some light stretching and calisthenic movements to get your heart pumping and your muscles loose. It's a way to transition your body from a cold (rested) state to a warmed-up (active) mode.

The purpose of the warm-up is to prepare your body for the real training that's coming up. The stretches should be performed slowly and steadily, and the exercise movements should be done correctly but at a low intensity. Deep stretching for flexibility should be done at the end of your session, when you're completely warmed up. If you're a person who is experienced in exercise, perform the warm-up that you like. Everyone's different; some need to do more or less than others. The important thing here is that you warm up your entire body. Appendix F shows the warm-up that I've used for many years. It's effective and takes about 5 minutes.

outs I've designed and use myself. One's for a gym that has a stair climber (or nearby stairs), another is a combo workout, and the other is a hike, really a Support workout.

I highly recommend that you wear boots (or at least very sturdy cross-training sneakers) when you do the weighted-vest sessions. Boots will protect your feet, and they have better support than running shoes for carrying that extra weight. Plus, most working people wear boots when they work. The problem is that most gyms won't let you wear boots in their gym, and I've been yelled at more than once for doing this. So if you're a firefighter and need to get some time on the stair climber machine, at least get some sturdy cross-trainers for that workout.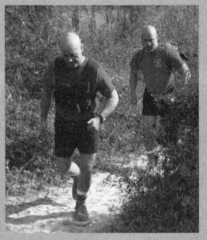

Again, not to try and sell you anything, but in my opinion the best boots for PT are Bates "Lites." They're very light and feel like running shoes, but provide the protection and support of boots. I must've run 1000 miles in Bates over the last ten years or so, and I feel they're a must for doing PT with boots. I try to do all my outside PT in boots (with or without a vest), and always try to do that training in the dirt, on the beach, or on grass (rather than on pavement). If I had my way, I'd wear nothing but these great boots for all my PT, but I have to wear running shoes/cross-trainers in the gym. To be honest, it also motivates the hell out of me. When I PT with boots, it just gets me in the right mindset instantly.

I also strongly recommend that you only do this type of weighted-vest training no more than once a week. This, along with actual work-related scenarios that'll come up and the rest of your training without the vest will be plenty. Doing tough training is a good thing, but breaking yourself before you even get to the fight is stupid. Train smart and you'll get in the right shape and keep your risk of injury to a minimum. Make sure you're listening to your half a brain.

Many experts, books, and magazines, will tell you that you need 15–20 minutes to warm up. Well, maybe for them, and maybe you need that also, but to be honest I normally don't have that much time just to warm up, nor have I ever found that I needed it. I've used this good 5-minute warm-up at 0400 on ice-cold mornings before PT, and I've NEVER had any injuries due to an improper warm-up. So, 5 minutes is enough for me.

Part 2. Pre-Fatigue (30 minutes)

It's been my experience that before you get to the actual point where you have to do something, you have to get there. Most of the time you have to get there fast, and with all your gear. A few practical examples: A firefighter may have to first climb up a long rescue ladder, carrying a heavy fire hose and wearing heavy protective equipment; then when he gets there he may have to hack through a door before dragging an injured person to safety. A police officer may have to chase a suspect for half a mile, and then wrestle him to the ground. A soldier may have to hump (hike) with a heavy pack several miles, drop his pack, run five blocks, and then become involved in a fire fight or even hand-to-hand combat. A roofer may have to carry dozens of bundles of heavy shingles up a ladder onto a roof, and then work all day laying the shingles. I can easily come up with 100 real-world examples of this.

The point is that in the real world you have to be able to think, act, and function when you're most likely already physically tired and mentally stressed. The only way you're going to learn to handle this for real is to practice it. Practice by progressively stressing your mind and body with a hard run, stair climb, bike ride, or similar repetitive movement before you do anything else. That's why you'll find that the Pre-Fatigue section is primarily endurance movements. It's to develop your aerobic ability, your ability to endure overall fatigue and stress. The time when you'll need to recover quickly and press on is when you're just about exhausted. It's in this "pre-fatigued" state that you'll need to be able to perform at your best, or at least hold it together. In real life, stressful situations rarely happen when you're fresh and well rested, or at regularly scheduled times.

In a nutshell, the purpose of Pre-Fatigue is to build up your wind/increase your lung power and develop your capacity to do repetitive tasks, and, as you might now guess, that's where it gets its name from. This can be done many ways, and you should pick the ones that target your fitness goals. If your goal is all-around fitness without any real specific requirement, you should use as many of the different movements as are practical, or just stick with a few you like best. There is almost no end to the different combinations you can come up with. Just stay within the guidelines of Pre-Fatigue and they'll all work.

Below is a list of some activities that are great for Pre-Fatigue sessions. Take your pick, thinking about your goals are and your situation (what equipment do you have, what's your location, weather conditions, etc.). Then try to stick with an exercise that will most closely prepare you for that task. In Appendix C, I've listed some sample Pre-Fatigue routines for you to try out. I encourage you to make up your own, too. I think of new ones all the time.

- Running (outside, or on a treadmill)
- Fast walking or hiking (humping) while wearing a weighted vest or pack, mixed in with short sprints
- Regular pedal bike or stationary bike (spinning bikes are best)
- Stair climber machine, or actual stairs
- Versa climber machine
- Elliptical or ski machine
- Rowing machine
- Skipping rope

I left out a bunch of things that can give you a serious endurance workout, like swimming, aerobics classes, spinning, etc. I left them out because they don't really provide the flexibility needed to fit into our time schedule. Swimming is a good example of why. If you take all the time and effort to get to a pool to swim, it's not practical to assume that you're going to swim for only 30 minutes, then get out, dry off, and change clothes just so you can lift weights and/or do calisthenics for 20 minutes. In a perfect circumstance I guess you could, but I set up this program to work in most cases, not exceptions. I'll talk about the right way to fit these activities into your overall schedule when I explain the "Support" part of all this later (page 46).

After your warm-up, pick one activity from the list and basically go as fast/hard as you can for a maximum of 30 minutes. There are an almost unlimited number of ways you can vary what you do within those 30 minutes, but the bottom line is that you have 30 minutes, so get busy.

Your present need/restriction in terms of schedule, energy level, location and available equipment will have a big impact on what you choose and how you actually conduct your 30 minutes. High-school running tracks, city/town parks, and playgrounds are all over the country. Many parks have running trails all marked out. In

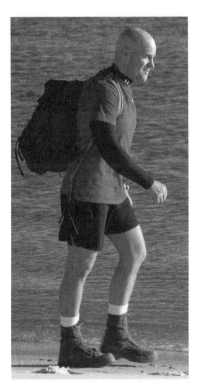

Appendix C, I lay out some basic Pre-Fatigue running workouts. These workouts can be done the same way on a treadmill, stationary bike, stair climber, or any of the machines I listed. You've got 30 minutes, and trust me: If you push yourself, you'll get all the lung power and Pre-Fatigue stress you'll ever need.

Within the Pre-Fatigue section (or any part of EPRS), you can go more slowly when you're tired and/or just starting out. Use that flexibility. You'll hear me stress constantly to increase the intensity of your PT, to get more done in the same amount of time. To get in better shape you have to push your body a little harder as you go so your body adapts to the stress. That's what being in better shape is all about: increasing your body's ability to handle physical and mental stress. But I'm not saying that you have to beat yourself into the ground, especially at first. I'm saying to slowly increase the intensity level of your PT to a point where you're feeling it but not killing yourself. Some boneheads (like me) like to push themselves to the point of puking when training, but it took me years to get to the point where I can do that without injuring myself. To get in great shape you have to push yourself hard, but get to that point at YOUR pace. Only you are in your body, so listen to yourself, push when you can, back off when you need to. Ignore the person on the treadmill, lifting weights, or running by you outside.

When your Pre-Fatigue portion is completed, move on to Mission with NO delay other than to take a drink of water and catch your breath. Real situations don't have built-in "time-outs." I realize that you'll have to build up slowly to a high intensity; however, keeping the right mindset is vital to make this work and get the most out of your limited time.

While I think that all of these Pre-Fatigue activities are good in their own way, I feel running, stair climbing, and humping (with or without a weighted vest) are the best overall for building working fitness. They're the most versatile and will yield you the biggest real benefits. They should always be your first choice if possible. However, I realize that not everyone likes running, stair climbing, and hiking as much as I do. I also realize that weather conditions are a factor. In many parts of the world, it's not practical (or safe) to PT outside year-round. That's why I include many different methods/movements for you to train with, both outside and in a gym. This allows you the flexibility to train hard in almost any circumstance. You could actually do a different movement every session. Again, this is your time. The point is to push yourself with one of these movements as hard as you can safely.

Part 3. Mission (20 minutes)

I call this section Mission to remind you of its purpose: that your training here is to help you complete a mission, whatever that may be. Pre-Fatigue got you here. Now you're a little tired, but you still have something to do. You have a mission. Get it?

Mission can be done in up to 20 minutes, or combined with the Pre-Fatigue section for 50 minutes total. Mission routines are specifically designed to build overall body power and the type of muscle strength that is needed for working fitness.

This is a good time to make a couple of points. First off, whether you're a man or woman, young or old, you need to be strong. Not just hard-ass-attitude wise, I mean physically strong. I realize that strength is a relative thing, as generally speaking men are naturally stronger than women (though not always; I've known some very strong women). Bigger people have the potential to be stronger than smaller people. That's simple physics. The development of overall body power and muscle strength is important to your health and well-being. This program will make you very strong.

Upping Your Intensity

Here are some ways to increase the intensity of the SAT:

- Move faster in your Pre-Fatigue section.
- Reduce your rest time between sets.
- Increase your reps.
- Increase your weights (about 50 percent of your body weight in any movement is all you'll need, but you can go higher if feel like it).

My definition of strength is the ability to apply muscular force in a focused manner, like chopping through a door with an axe, loading hundreds of sandbags, or doing pull-ups. It can also be defined as physical toughness, like the strength that it takes to hike 20 miles with a heavy pack, or the ability to do grueling manual work for many hours.

Power is your body's ability to move other objects, like heavy gear or another person, or crashing through a locked door. Simply speaking, it's the application of brute force. Having one doesn't mean you have the other. I have known some Marines who could run through a brick wall but couldn't do three good pull-ups. The bottom line is that you need a balance of both power and strength to really be physically fit. (Yes, I realize that these definitions aren't scientific, but you should get my drift here, genius.)

A bigger person can naturally have more power as they're pushing or pulling from a heavier base. That doesn't mean a small person can't have a ton of power, though. I've seen it myself. I spent the majority of my Marine Corps career working in Aviation Ordnance. This can be one of the most physically challenging career fields in the military. Just about every task consists of the repetitive physical movement of very heavy pieces of explosive ordnance and support equipment. People doing this have to be very strong for their body weight, and have to work as a team to load 500- to 2000-pound bombs onto aircraft, trailers, etc. At times, this has to be done around the clock, at a very hectic pace, and it doesn't matter if it's on the rolling flight deck of a Navy ship, or in 120-degree heat in Iraq. It takes training, leadership, and teamwork to move these extremely heavy pieces of ordnance around on time without people getting injured. It's a real test of "working fitness." Years of doing this myself and observing my Marines working during these hectic work periods also helped me develop my system.

Make no mistake, however. Our mission here is not body building. While you'll definitely improve your appearance as you lose fat and condition your body. The purpose of EPRS is to develop a "go" body, not a "show" body. If your only goal is to develop a large, heavily muscled physique, this is not the system for you. EPRS will bring your body to a place where it performs at its best (long term), and that includes your actual weight. For 99 percent of the world, that isn't the build of Mr. America, power lifter or pro football player. Think more of the look of a boxer, college wrestler, track athlete, or even a professional bull rider. The point being is that it's more important that form follows function, not the other way around.

While I'm on this "looks vs. performance" subject, let me address another popular thing. It's the infamous six-pack abs. Listen, I've seen homeless alcoholics who had a nice set of abs. The whole "ab" thing is mostly a matter of body fat content, nothing else, so like huge biceps, it's not a great indicator of real fitness. If you're seriously injured in a car accident and a firefighter or a cop has to get you to safety, do you care if he has a six pack? If you need to carry your children or spouse from a burning house or car, do you think six-pack abs will be on your mind? I seriously doubt it. Having six-pack abs won't make any difference in life-saving situations. Being able to perform in the real world is the purpose of EPRS.

The strength and power-training part of SAT is done with a combination of weights and calisthenics. When speaking of weights I'm talking about dumbbells and/or kettlebells. In my opinion, a combination of calisthenics and dumbbell/kettlebell weights works the best for building the kind of strength and power you need for working fitness. You can use barbells, but I think dumbbells and, especially, kettlebells are better overall. If you have any experience in lifting weights, you know that lifting the same amount of weight on a barbell is easier than with two dumbbells of equal weight, and kettlebells are even harder. It's because they require both hands to do equal work, meaning you need more balance and a stronger grip to do the same work. Also kettlebells and dumbbells are more portable. This is an important consideration as you can take them almost anywhere and do PT. (For more about dumbbells and kettlebells, see Training Tips on page 40.)

I've competed in Olympic-style and power-lifting competitions, and lifted some pretty heavy weights in my day. Without a doubt lifting weights is the best way to build overall body power and muscle strength. While I'll spare you the details of all my sub-heroic lifting feats, I will say that my best overall lift was probably when I was 18 and training in the Olympic style. One day in the gym I made a very sloppy power clean and jerk of 235 pounds at a body weight of around 140 pounds. Maybe that doesn't sound like that much to some, but nobody, including some pretty big guys, in the big, crowded gym I was in could do it. To this day I look at 235 pounds on a bar and wonder how my scrawny ass ever got that much over my head. I wouldn't try it now. I only throw that out there to show that I've gone pretty heavy at times myself so I have some insight into what the negative and positive aspects of lifting heavy are.

While lifting very heavy in all the standard lifts (bench press, squats, overhead press, dead lifts, etc.), I found that my ability to lift heavy weights in itself had very little to do with improving my overall fitness. I was always sore, my joints ached, and I had a hard time keeping my body weight down. While I was very strong in all the lifts, that's all I seemed to really improve in. When I look back now at it honestly, it never seemed to add much to my overall condition. I've also known many people who trained with very heavy weights. Not all were huge guys—many were smaller guys who were just very strong people. I observed that almost all of them (of any size) had some serious knee, shoulder, and/or back problems.

Having said all that, it's my experience that lifting very heavy weights is not necessary to build working fitness, and in most cases will not help you get into the condition you really need. Other than for certain sports like football, body building, or actual weight-lifting competitions, its benefits are not worth the risk of injuries (both long- and short-term) that are sure to come. For the purposes of working fitness, going heavy is not needed or recommended. As a general guideline, lifting around 50 percent of your actual body weight is all you need to get and stay in some very serious condition. I know a lot of people will strongly disagree with me on this (I've heard it for years) but time and time again my observation and experience have proven this to be the way to go.

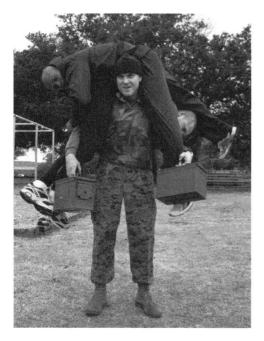

Look at it from a practical standpoint: Nowadays I weigh in at about 165 pounds. Fifty percent of that is approximately 85 pounds, or roughly two 40- or 45-pound dumbbells or kettlebells. The vast majority of real-life activities are not going to require me to lift more than that. What real-world situations *will* call for is the ability to lift, move, and carry that weight (and your butt) over and over—over hills, up stairs, over sand, up and down ladders, etc. If there's a situation where you have to move a very heavy weight, say 200+ pounds, you'll be able to handle it, meaning you'll be able to move it a short distance with little trouble, or more likely be able to hold up your end working with others to move it. I haven't trained with heavy weights in years, but if you'll note the picture to your left, you'll see me wearing a flak jacket and carrying two guys and two ammo cans—a combined total weight of over 400 pounds at a body weight of around 165 pounds—without any problem.

For another example, when I was working construction we would pour concrete basement floors. This was always done as the house was being built, or even after it was completed. What you have to do is back the concrete truck up to one of the little basement windows and pour the concrete down a shoot into the basement. The rub here is that they can't always get the truck around to but one or two spots, meaning that down inside the basement you have to spread the concrete by the shovelful around the floor. While a shovel full of concrete probably only weighs about 10 pounds or so (and unless you want to get the nickname of "Teaspoon" you always take a full shovel's worth), you may have to sling that shovel 1,000 times or more to get the job done. That's with very little rest to catch your breath. You have to move quickly because as you're working the concrete starts to set. This is just another example of the kind of physical conditioning you need in the real world.

The Exercise Glossary (pages 81–99) is a picture index with basic instructions on all the exercises I recommend. I've tried hundreds of different types of calisthenics and weightlifting movements, and just about every exercise/weightlifting machine found in a gym. I only list the ones I feel are the most effective for this program.

Over time I've spent many hours developing Mission sessions. I've done so because I knew this would be a very important part of obtaining the fitness level I was looking for. To get it right I tested many different combinations of movements to get the most effective results in the shortest amount of time.

34   CORPS STRENGTH

Before I give you some sample Mission workouts and take you through one, we need to go over a few things so you understand the thought process that led to this system. I've grouped movements in cycles as I found this is the best way to generate the balanced intensity required to develop working fitness. Utilizing a balanced whole-body approach conditions the right areas in the right way. Splitting up exercises by isolating body parts, in my opinion, is a mistake. That type of program was designed years ago by body builders to isolate muscle groups in order to promote their maximum growth. I'm sure you've heard the common biceps/back, chest/triceps stuff before. I used to do it myself. It's a great method for its designed purpose (looks), but not a good idea for working fitness. Muscle groups that move together must be trained together for high performance. In fact, it's been my experience and observation that this type of isolation training will lead to an imbalance in how your body interacts and, eventually, injury.

In Mission sessions, the cycles are designed to be performed in a specific order to maximize your time, effort, and results. All sessions are broken down the same basic way: 3 cycles of 3 rotations, 2 exercises each, and 1 cycle of 2 rotations, 2 exercises each.

This probably sounds way more complicated than it is, but once you do it a few times, it's a no-brainer.

Cycle 1   Pull-up/Push-ups: 1 set of pull-ups rotated with 1 set of push-ups, 3X
Cycle 2   Wheel-house/Abs: A set of wheel-house movements rotated with a set of abs, 3X
Cycle 3   Assist/Abs: A set of assist movements rotated with a set of abs, 3X
Cycle 4   Grip-Neck/Abs: A set of grip or neck movements rotated with one set on abs in between, 2X

Cycle 1> Pull-ups/Push-ups   These should always be performed first because they're basic conditioning movements. They're also non-weightlifting movements that will provide the right transition from your mostly aerobic Pre-Fatigue session into the mostly weightlifting Mission session. The pull-up is not only very important but a tough exercise that needs to done while you're still relatively fresh. Pull-ups are rotated with push-ups to provide the right balance between pulling and pushing movements.

Cycle 2> Wheel-house/Abs   Wheel-house movements are exercises that target the "wheel-house" area of your body—basically your legs, hips, lower back, and butt, where the largest and most powerful muscles in your body hang out. Simply put, it's roughly the area of your body from your knees to your belly button. To be working fit, your wheel-house must be strong, flexible, and injury free. When I'm training people in boxing I always stress that real punching power comes from your wheel-house, not from your arms. The same can be said about any body movement that requires power and long-term endurance—everything from sports, like hitting a baseball, to pure physical labor, like loading heavy boxes of hurricane supplies onto a truck, or hiking with a heavy pack. Your wheel-house is where real working fitness comes from.

These movements train these muscles to work together to develop power and conditioning. They'll also get your breathing up as they're good aerobically. Wheel-house movements are rotated with abs to keep up the intensity and to balance out the cycle.

Cycle 3> Assist/Abs   Assist/Abs exercises are movements that "assist" in your conditioning program, conditioning your wheel-house more than anything else. As the Master of the Obvious I need to point out that your arms and shoulders will never be as strong as your legs, but you need strong arms and shoulders to be able to

Calisthenics

Some time or other you'll probably find yourself someplace or in a situation where you don't have access to any type of weights. In this case you'll only have the ability to do calisthenics for your Mission session. My feeling on this is that while you can stay in pretty decent shape with only calisthenics, without some type of extra weight to condition your body, you'll never really get into top condition.

This will raise some eyebrows as there are many calisthenics-only programs out there, but the reason is simple. Calisthenic programs work only with your body weight, but military members, first responders, and most working people simply don't do anything without their gear, whether they're wearing it or carrying it. That's the bottom line on this, and it's one of the big reasons I designed my system to always utilize weights if possible. However, I'll say that for certain occupations, a routine that has no weights may be the way to go. These are occupations that require heavy lifting day in and day out, such as masons, longshoremen, loading dock personnel, lumberjacks, etc. They probably get enough of a lifting workout in their everyday routine, so their focus should be aerobic conditioning and flexibility—a non-weight/calisthenic program would be the way to go for them.

Having said all that, keep in mind that a weight is something heavy that you can pick up. I've done Mission-type workouts with sandbags, logs, ammo cans, tool boxes, large rocks, big tires, beer kegs, tie-down chains, buckets of sand, and even bowling balls. Look around and use your imagination. If you have to use one of these odd items, just try and simulate the Mission weightlifting movements as closely as you can.

When I was stationed in New Orleans, we got one of those huge bucket-loader tires from a junkyard and flipped it around at the end of every workout. It was great for overall body power and fun to do, but it's not really a practical training tool for the average person, as it was about six feet across and weighed in at about

hold on to and position objects (including your own body weight) that your wheel-house is going to move around. A different series of ab movements are rotated with the assist exercises.

Cycle 4> Grip or Neck/Abs   Mission always ends with a Grip/Neck cycle. This cycle is done for only two rotations, with a final single abdominal movement performed in between. Grip and especially neck conditioning are two of the most overlooked areas of physical fitness. You need to do grip or neck conditioning at the end of every Mission workout in an alternating manner so that you do neck one workout and grip the next.

I have good reason for this. Keeping your neck strong and flexible has many benefits, not the least of which is to help keep your back injury free. A strong neck is needed to support heavy protective headgear and, of course, help you absorb impact to your head—not just for sports like boxing or football but in everyday life. A few years back in New Orleans, some butthole ran a stoplight and totaled my new truck (a year's worth of saved combat pay went to the junkyard). The collision was pretty rough, and I smacked my grape right into the windshield (the airbag didn't come out). I cracked the windshield and got a nice bump on my forehead, but other than that I didn't even have a headache. I'm convinced my well-conditioned neck helped keep me from serious injury (my strong neck didn't help get my truck fixed, however).

400 pounds. However, if you can get one and have a place to use it, go ahead. Funny thing about that tire, when I was a kid working at the gravel pit, I had to move big tires like that one around all the time for my job. But back then it was called work, not exercise.

If you have your weight vest, you're good to go since you could wear it for your Mission session instead of using weights. Still, don't try and run with it every workout—only once a week at the most, as I recommended earlier. If you don't have anything you can use for weights, here are two calisthenics-only Mission workouts you can use with or without a vest. These are done with three movements per cycle to up the intensity. For the pull-ups and push-ups, rotate through them all or do them in a manner like the abs (doing a different one each set). What if you don't have anywhere to do pull-ups? Work with your lawyer for an early release.

Calisthenics-Only Mission Workout 1
> *Cycle 1* Any pull-up (10X3), next any push-up (25X3), next abs A, B, C (50 ea)
>
> *Cycle 2* Free Squats (25X3), next Mountain Climbers (25X3), next abs D, E, F (50 ea)

Calisthenics-Only Mission Workout 2
> *Cycle 1* Any pull-up (10X3), next any push-up (25X3), next abs A, B, C (50 ea)
>
> *Cycle 2* Step-ups (10X3), next 8 counts (10X3), next abs D, E, F (50 ea)

For these programs, complete Cycle 1 (do one set of pull-ups, one set of push-ups, abs A x50, then another set of pull-ups, another set of push-ups, abs B x50, then a final set of pull-ups, a final set of push-ups, abs C x50) before moving on to Cycle 2.

In the Mission section, when you see "Neck," just do whatever neck movement you like (see Appendix B, pages 92–93) or can do. Try to mix them up. I like neck bridges the best, but I'll admit these are tough to do on anything but a mat of some type. When doing PT outside of a gym, you may not have the ability to do a neck workout. You can, but it isn't practical to do neck bridges on the bare ground or concrete, even with a towel. What works better for when you're outside (and it works just as well inside) is a neck harness. You can buy it at any local sporting goods store. With that you can attach your dumbbell or kettlebell to it and you're in business. It's also easy to travel with. If you don't have one and you're doing a Mission session outside, just stick with doing grip movements until you can get a harness or when you're back in a place where you can work your neck properly. The most important thing about neck training is to go slowly, lightly, and carefully. I've been doing neck bridges for over 30 years without a problem; however, most people, even those who exercise regularly, don't do anything for their neck. So start VERY slowly and go easy. It's probably also the easiest part of your body to injure if you try to do too much. You've been warned.

The need for grip strength speaks for itself. You need a strong grip to do almost anything. A strong grip could save your life, as you may have to hang on to keep from falling—ask any firefighter or construction worker who has worked off the ground. I've always been impressed with a strong grip. My dad is over 70 years old and has worked with his hands all his life. He startles people with his very strong handshake. His brother, my uncle Bud, used to work for the phone company splicing cables together. He had a pair of small, very stout "lineman's scissors" that he worked with all day long cutting wires and small cables. When I was a kid, I once watched him (after he had drunk a few beers) cut a coin in half with those things, and it wasn't because the scissors were bolt cutters. It was because he had a grip like a vise.

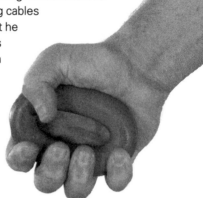

I've used many different types of grippers over the years, but nowadays I use a rock climber's "doughnut" made by Grip Pro Trainer. This solid rubber doughnut-shaped gripper can be squeezed like any other gripper of this type, but what makes this one better is that you can stick your fingers inside the hole and also work your finger strength by pushing out. As you know, rock climbers cram their fingers into holes in a cliff face and support their body weight. I think they're nuts, but they have some serious grip/hand strength. I have three of these dough-nuts: in my car, in my home, and in my bag for when I travel. It's a good piece of gear and doesn't cost squat.

Your grip gets a workout in almost every other movement in my system, so it only needs relatively little direct exercise. However, this must be very intense because we use our gripping muscles so much in everyday life that it's a tough group of muscles to really fatigue. You need to do a high number of repetitions to get condition-ing. Two rotations of a maximum number of reps is the way to go for grip conditioning. The bottom line is you need to condition your neck and work your grip.

Some sample Mission workouts are listed on the facing page. All of them have been designed to be equally effective for your entire body. They should be performed in the order I have laid out. Six can be done almost anywhere, and the last one (Mission 7) you need a gym. I do all of these, and they're all good. After you do them all, you'll find two or three you like best and will do those more often (I like 1 and 4 best), but do them all for vari-ety and balance. You can come up with an almost endless number of different routines yourself. Just pick the exercises from each section (see the Exercise Glossary on pages 81–99) and plug them into the right sequence. Or you may just want to stick with these—but make sure to perform the right sequence. They're all balanced, effective, and will fit in your time frame.

I've listed numbers of repetitions for each exercise as goals for you to work toward. With some effort, you can easily reach all these rep goals, and it can all be done in 20 minutes or less. You can actually do much more, but it ain't easy; you'll have to kick it. Depending on where you are or what gear you have, you may have to adjust your routine slightly. But if you have access to a place where you have something to do pull-ups on, a set of dumbbells/kettlebells, you can do all of these workouts without a problem: in a gym or outside at most parks or high school tracks.

Let's go over Mission 1 together just so we're on the same page. First, start with a set of regular pull-ups, fol-lowed by a set of regular push-ups—that's one rotation. Without any more rest than you need, repeat this two more times. That's one cycle. Then move on to cycle 2, which is deadlift curls and abs A, B, and C. Once you've finished that, do cycle 3: overhead press and abs D, E, F. Finish with cycle 4: two sets of grip exercise with a single set of abs G in between. Like I said, it's not hard to figure out once you get the basic flow down.

Sample Missions

Mission 1 *Cycle 1* Regular Pull-ups (10X3), alternating with Regular Push-ups (25X3)

Cycle 2 Deadlift Curls (10–15X3), alternating with Abs A, B, C (50 ea)

Cycle 3 Overhead Press (10–15x3), alternating with Abs D, E, F (50 ea)

Cycle 4 Grip (Max X2), alternating with Abs G (50)

Mission 2 *Cycle 1* Chin-ups (10X3), alternating with Wide Push-ups (25X3)

Cycle 2 Step-up Shrugs (10–15X3), alternating with Abs B, C, D (50 ea)

Cycle 3 Triceps Press (10–15X3), alternating with Abs E, F, G (50 ea)

Cycle 4 Neck (X2), alternating with Abs A (50)

Mission 3 *Cycle 1* Close-grip Pull-ups (10X3), alternating with Diamond Push-ups (25X3)

Cycle 2 Squat Press (10–15X3), alternating with Abs C, D, E (50 ea)

Cycle 3 Upright Rows (10–15X3), alternating with Abs F, G, A (50 ea)

Cycle 4 Grip (Max X2), alternating with Abs B (50)

Mission 4 *Cycle 1* Behind-the-neck Pull-ups (10X3), alternating with Incline Push-ups (25X3)

Cycle 2 Lateral Swings (10–15X3), alternating with Abs D, E, F (50 ea)

Cycle 3 Hammer Curls (10–15X3), alternating with Abs G, A, B (50 ea)

Cycle 4 Neck (X2), alternating with Abs C (50)

Mission 5 *Cycle 1* Commando Pull-ups (10–15X3), alternating with Mountain Climber Push-ups (5–10X3)

Cycle 2 Farmer Walk (20 yardsX3), alternating with Abs E, F, G (50 ea)

Cycle 3 Rows (10–15X3), alternating with Abs A, B, C (50 ea)

Cycle 4 Grip (Max X2), alternating with Abs D (50)

Mission 6 *Cycle 1* V-ups (10X3), alternating with Regular Push-ups (25X3)

Cycle 2 Front Squats (5–10X3), alternating with Abs F, G, A (50 ea)

Cycle 3 Front Raises (10–15X3), alternating with Abs B, C, D (50 ea)

Cycle 4 Neck (X2), alternating with Abs E (50)

Mission 7 *Cycle 1* Pull-down machine (15–20X3), alternating with Dips (25X3)

Cycle 2 Cable Row machine (15–20X3), alternating with Abs G, A, B (50 ea)

Cycle 3 Cable Upright Row (15–20X3), alternating with Abs C, D, E (50 ea)

Cycle 4 Grip (Max X2), alternating with Abs F (50)

I could've listed many more movements here, but I listed the ones I think are the most effective. I left out all the ones I don't like, like lunges, for example. Over the years I tried lots of lunges, and no matter how I did them they always made my knees hurt. I know many experts will swear by them, but I won't recommend anything to anyone that I won't do myself. The same goes for all the popular "planks." You know those static hold-in-place exercises? This program is designed to enhance your movement, not your ability to hold still. Never got those, and don't do them or recommend them.

It's also the reason that I left out pretty much all the traditional weightlifting movements such as bench press and barbell squat. While it would be easy to fill up a workout guide with these exercises, I simply think they're overrated to achieve working fitness. First off, life's contests must be dealt with from the ground up, meaning that the most likely challenges of your strength, power, and endurance will be performed on your feet. The effective movements to prepare for these are performed as such, or in a manner that simulates real-body movements. Lying on your back and pushing a weight up doesn't translate into many practical real-life requirements that I know of. Other than in bench pressing for competition or trying to build a large chest, it has little actual benefit. I stay away from almost all weightlifting machines for the same reason. They lock your body into an unnatural position to isolate a muscle—not something that will develop working fitness.

Strengthening your abdominal region (your core) is also very important. Just about everything you do in moving your body involves your midsection in one way or the other. A strong midsection is also important in helping to keep your back, especially your lower back, healthy. In this program, I almost always integrate abdominal movements between other movements. It's a great way to keep your intensity level up, and a very effective way to fit more exercise into a shorter time period. To me it also seems to balance out the workout. While there are many different abdominal movements you can do. I like the seven exercises featured in this book the best, as they can be done anywhere and will keep your abs in great shape. (See pages 97–99 for instruction on the abdominal movements.) In the Mission cycles, rotate all seven ab movements for each workout, and change the order each time to make it harder.

Training Tips
Here are some tips that'll make your workouts much more efficient and effective.

Weight Training
When doing movements that utilize dumbbells or kettlebells, use a weight that gets you in the 10–15 rep range. This should be easy enough to do at a gym that has dumbbells in all different sizes. If you're using your own fixed set and you consistently can do over 15 reps (like 20 fairly easy), consider purchasing the next step up in weight. For instance, I'd been using a set of 30-pound kettlebells; when those started to feel light, I moved up to a pair of 40 pounders. That feels like a much bigger leap than it sounds, as I've tried them out already, and it'll probably be a long time before I move up again, if ever. Because of the way you lift kettlebells, they feel heavier than dumbbells. In addition to a set of kettlebells of equal weight, I have a single kettlebell that is 62 pounds. I use this for deadlifts, rows, and overhead presses. It can be a monster in certain movements, and doing a movement with a single heavy kettlebell vs. two lighter ones puts a different spin on your conditioning.

While they're somewhat expensive (roughly twice the cost of the same-size solid dumbbell), I highly recommend buying a set of kettlebells. These are the closest thing you can get to a portable gym. I always take mine on any trip that requires me to drive. Before I became aware of kettlebells several years ago, I used (and still have) a pair of solid 40-pound dumbbells. They're still good enough, but I think kettlebells are better, as they're harder to deal with and are more versatile. (The 40-pound kettlebells also feel heavier than the 40-pound dumbbells.) They're a great investment, require no maintenance, and are just about indestructible, meaning they'll last many years of hard use. For what you can get out of them, they're worth much more than what they cost. If you just get a pair that together are about half your weight, you'll be good to go for every movement I've listed. Add to that a weighted vest as well as a neck harness, and you have just about everything you need to get into some serious condition almost anywhere, and at the time of your choosing. The total cost of those items will be much less than any of those home fitness gizmos you see advertised 24/7 on TV, and they're much more effective and will last much longer.

You could also get a couple of ammo cans from the local military surplus store. If you get a standard-size ammo can (.50 cal machine gun ammo can), filling it with sand will make it weigh about 30 pounds; you can add some small weight plates in with the sand and make them much heavier if you want to. This is a very inexpensive but useful piece of gear. It has its limits (the handles can break off, they're difficult to do certain exercises with), but it can be used for most exercises. I like the fact that they're somewhat awkward to handle, which in itself is training. Plus there's something that's motivating about throwing some ammo cans around, and motivation should never be disregarded.

Pull-Ups

If you're doing your PT in a well-outfitted gym, I recommend that you substitute the lat pull-down machine for pull-ups once a week, especially on days when you're feeling a little tired. It breaks thing up, and it's a good way to help you increase your pull-up ability. You should also do cable rows (upright and flat). These cable moves are very effective, as they provide constant tension throughout the movements, just like when you're actually pulling something toward you in a real situation, like lifting or pulling something up with a rope. When doing these machine movements, pick a weight that keeps you in a slightly higher rep range of 15–20 as it's the best opportunity to help develop the high end of your pull-up (pulling) range. Pull-ups are tough, but they're an important fundamental exercise to achieve working fitness, and the reason we always do them first.

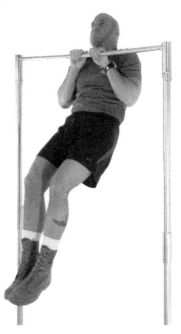

Some gyms have a pull-up machine, which gives you a weight assist to help you build strength (more reps) in pull-ups. It's a good piece of gear if you have trouble getting five good pull-ups. If you can do 3 sets of 5 strict pull-ups, you really don't need it. Just keep at it. It may be slow going, but you'll get better. (In the Exercise Glossary on page 85, I show how a friend or chair can assist you in getting a few extra when you can't get any more.) On pull-ups, 10 reps may not seem like a hard goal for some of you, or too much for others. What I find is that 3 sets of 10 reps is about right for behind-the-neck pull-ups. I can easily do more of the others, but I think 10 is a good baseline goal for all of them. If 10 is too easy, just do as many as you can—don't stop at 10. If you can't do 10, just get what you can. It's a goal, remember. Make sure you watch your form, go all the way down, and don't "kip" (swing your body excessively to help you get over the bar).

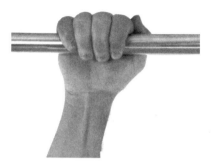

Another thing about pull-ups is your grip. Don't oppose your thumb— just grasp the bar with your four fingers and put your thumb on the same side. This will feel weird at first, especially if you're used to doing them the other way. There are a couple of advantages to this. First, if you don't oppose your grip, the thickness of the bar will have little effect on how many you can do. When you grip the normal way, the thickness of the bar can have an effect. Trust me on this one, I didn't believe it at first. A Navy SEAL that I used to box with showed me this, and he was right. Once you get used to it, it's worth at least one or two more in a max set. The only time that wrapping your thumb around the bar is an advantage is on a very thin bar, which in my experience is something you run across very infrequently. What normally happens is bars will get thicker and thicker as some genius is always putting more tape around them. The other advantage is that your grip is less likely to tire out before you max out your pull-ups.

For years I used to do a lot of pyramid sets for pull-ups. You may be familiar with some of those routines. It's where you do a step-up series of reps like: 1-2-3-4-5-4-3-2-1. I stopped as my system was coming together. While I (and others I trained) had some decent success with this "step" method, I eventually switched to a system of more reps and less sets (with a few assisted reps at the end of each set). The step method didn't work very well for what I was trying to do (or train others to do), which was to get 20 reps on the Marine Corps PFT. The tough part of that test is reps 15–20. To get better at that range, you have to spend more time on the bar— more reps, in other words. I also like to do a max set the first set when I'm fresh; this gives you a better idea of your actual condition as you're training. I never liked having my max set in the middle after I had already performed several lower-rep sets to get to it. Plus the step method can take a long time to do. Once in a while I still do some pyramid sets to break things up, but overall I think more reps, lower sets is the way to go.

Part 4: Cool-Down (5 minutes)

The last part of the SAT is 5 minutes of cool-down and stretching. This is where you work on your flexibility and let your muscles cool down. You should be able to do a good stretch and cool-down in roughly 5 minutes. It's important that you always stretch at the end when you're warm. It'll make you less sore the next day, and being more flexible overall has many benefits, including making you less susceptible to injury. In Appendix G (page 112), I outline a cool-down and stretch routine that I use and recommend. It takes about 5 minutes.

Recap

Here's a PT session I did recently: Since the weather was good to go, I went to a local Navy base where they had a standard quarter-mile track with pull-up bars nearby. Wearing boots, shorts, and a T-shirt (my favorite PT uniform), I took my two 40-pound kettlebells with me. I completed my normal warm-up, and then, for the Pre-Fatigue section, I jogged a half mile to loosen up, then sprinted the straight-aways and jogged the turns. I alternated sprinting/jogging till I got 3 miles, finishing in just over 27 minutes. (As a note when running, I always stop at 3 miles if I can get to it before 30 minutes. I push myself to finish 3 miles in less than 30 minutes, and 99 percent of the time I do, normally finishing around 26–27 minutes. That's around an 8:30-mile average run, which may be too fast for some and too slow for others, but either way, when running I use that 3-mile mark as an incentive. I feel this is a very reasonable goal for a healthy person. I usually go slow at first to warm up, and gradually speed up and finish the last mile pretty fast, especially the last quarter mile. A few times when I was feeling very tired, I didn't get to 3 miles in 30 minutes. This only happened a few times, but it's no biggie. As I told you in the beginning, the times are a guideline to help you keep your intensity up. You aren't going to be able to go all out every PT session. You have good days and bad days. The point here is to push hard when you feel good, back off a little when you don't. If you're doing things the right way, you'll have many more good days than bad overall. A day you get to PT is a good day in any case, as far as I'm concerned.)

Right after my run I got a drink of water and went over to the pull-up bars next to the running track. As you know, with Mission we always start with a pull-up/push-up cycle. They're primary strength builders and are a good way to lead into lifting any actual weights. I decided to do Mission 1 with kettlebells (I list the actual reps I got for instructional purposes):

> 3 sets of Regular Pull-ups, alternating with Regular Push-ups.
> Totals: Pull-ups 22, 16, 13. Regular push-ups 40, 35, 30
> *(When I say alternating I mean a set of pull-ups, THEN a set of push-ups.*
> *Catch your breath and do the cycle two more times).*

Next: 3 sets of Kettlebell Deadlift Curls, alternating with Abs movements A, B, C.
Totals: Deadlift Curls 10, 11, 12. Abs 50, 50, 50

Next: 3 Sets of Kettlebell Overhead Presses, alternating with Abs movements D, E, F
Totals: Overhead Presses 10, 10, 11. Abs 50, 50, 50

Next: 2 sets of Kettlebell Wrist Curls with one set of Abs G in between.
Totals: Wrist Curls max, max. Abs 50

I stretched out for about 5 minutes and was finished in 57 minutes.

That's 57 minutes to do:

- A good warm-up
- 3-mile run in just over 27 minutes
- 51 regular pull-ups
- 105 regular push-ups
- 33 kettlebell deadlift curls
- 31 kettlebell overhead presses
- 2 sets max kettlebell wrist curls
- 350 abdominal counts
- A good stretch and cool-down.

That's 57 minutes of almost continuous movement during which I worked myself in every area—strength, endurance, and flexibility—from head to toe. In the end I also had 3 minutes left. Next time I'll add some reps to all the movements and try to run faster (good luck).

I have my reasons for organizing things the way I have. The bottom line is I've worked through all of these SAT sessions in all different combinations, dozens of times, for years now. I'm not saying that I've tried every possible combination, but I have done more than I can remember. Try and make up some of your own. I know that these work, and all fit in the time guidelines IF you push it the way you should. While it may seem a little complicated at first, trust me—this isn't rocket science. If you can remember all the passwords, PIN numbers, and phone numbers you have, you can remember this stuff with no problem. Or you can do what I do and write it down. I have a Day Runner that I use for work. On the calendar part I simply write a few words here and there about what I did. I don't write down all the exercises, sets, and reps. I only did that above to give you an idea of the total work that was done. Any more than a few notes and to me it would become a pain in the rear to keep up. However, I know a lot of people who like to write detailed entries about their PT. If that's your thing, go ahead. Otherwise, it's easy stuff to remember once you do it a few times. Now that's the basics of SAT.

The intensity level is based on your present fitness level. To reduce the intensity of the session I described above, you could do a number of things: jog the straights and walk the turns; use a much lighter set of kettlebells; do less reps in each calisthenic; rest a little longer in between. Use the structure of the system but adjust the weights, reps, and exercises to your needs and your fitness levels. I can't stress this enough. Use the system to achieve your individual fitness needs.

SAT is the heart of my system and needs to be performed for at least half of your 3–5 hours a week that you've set aside for PT. I've laid out the way to schedule SAT and Support (I'll cover Support shortly on page 46) sessions over a seven-day cycle below. I didn't say a weekly schedule as the actual days of the cycle are up to you.

 3 sessions> SAT-Off-Sup-Off-SAT-Off-Off

 4 sessions> SAT-Sup-Off-SAT-Sup-Off-Off

 5 sessions> SAT-Sup-Off-SAT-Sup-SAT(or)Sup-Off

 6 sessions> SAT-Sup-SAT-Sup-SAT-Sup-Off

To make it simple, you could also just go SAT-Sup every other day. Keeping it simple is always good.

Combos

On the days that you're feeling "froggy" (meaning you have plenty of energy), you should combine the Pre-Fatigue and Mission sessions for about 50 minutes of non-stop movement. I call it a "combo." When done with high intensity (speed and very little rest), this can be a real ass kicker. Even at lower levels of intensity, it's a great way to break up your routine and try something new. I normally replace any standard SAT workout with a combo two to three times a month. This is also one you can do with a partner or partners easily. With combos, it helps to have the motivation that a partner can bring. Here are some examples of how to do this:

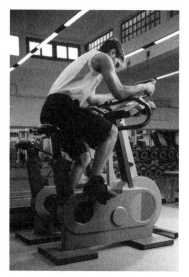

In a Gym
Warm-up (5 minutes): Treadmill 1 mile as fast as possible.

Next: 3 sets of any pull-ups, alternating with any push-ups.

Next: Stationary Bike 1 mile as fast as possible.

Next: 3 sets any wheel-house movement, alternating with any ab movement.

44 CORPS STRENGTH

Next: Stair Climber 5 minutes as fast as possible.

Next: 3 sets any assist movement, alternating with any ab movement

Next: Skip rope 5 minutes, with 10 push-ups every time you miss.

Stretch out and cool down 5 minutes.

That brings you to about an hour. If you can do all that without much effort, you're in serious shape and don't need me to tell you how to PT.

Outside Combo

You can use ammo cans, dumbbells, or kettlebells in any open field or big yard where you have something you can do pull-ups on.

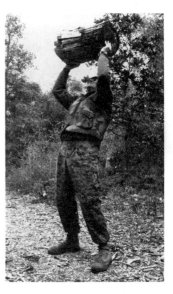

(Note your watch.)

Warm-up (5 minutes)

Start at where you're going to do pull-ups.

Pick up the ammo cans and jog or walk about 25 yards down the field.

Stop and do a set of push-ups.

Pick up the ammo cans and go back to the pull-up bars.

Do a set of pull-ups.

Pick up the ammo cans and jog or walk about 25 yards down the field.

Do a set of overhead presses with one can.

Pick up the ammo cans and go back to the pull-up bars.

Do a set of pull-ups.

Repeat this rotation with a different ammo can movement, calisthenic, pull-up, or push-up till you get to 50 minutes on your watch—50 minutes of this non-stop can seem like 50 hours. Then do your normal stretch/cooldown for 5 minutes.

The bottom line is that you can make combos as tough as you can handle. This is one PT session that works great for a group of people, and there's almost no end to the different routines you could do. Use your imagination.

CHAPTER 5

SUPPORT

SAT is the core of this system, and that's all you really need to do to stay in great shape. It'll become a no-brainer after you do it for awhile. However, your overall conditioning and attitude will be better if you don't do just SAT. SAT can be enhanced by what I call "Support," which means exactly that. It supports the SAT workout by adding variety and different types of exercise intensity. In a nutshell, Support training is an exercise/activity that is singular in nature. It could be:

- Long-distance running
- Cross-country skiing
- Backpacking, hiking
- Basketball
- Boxing, karate, judo, or MMA
- Scuba, snorkeling, free diving
- Military unit PT or unit training that is physical, like humping a pack, obstacle course
- Swimming
- Mountain biking or road cycling
- Rock climbing
- Motocross, off-road dirt bike riding
- Racquetball, handball, tennis, volleyball, hockey (in-line or ice)
- Spinning or aerobics class

In other words, it's any activity or sport that is strenuous and done for at least an hour. You could add splitting wood or shoveling snow to that list. I think you get the idea. I know I left some good stuff off the list, but give me a break, I can't list everything. The rule of thumb here is if you're not breathing hard and sweating after 5–10 minutes, it's not really Support. Lying on the beach is not swimming; walking around the block is not hiking. Get the picture? The plan with this is simple: You need to do this one or two times a week for at least an hour. Support can be good for the weekends and days off, and can last a few hours to all day long (like hiking, for example). My normal thing is to get in one long run of five miles or so a week and do something more fun (sports) the other time.

If you're a weekend athlete, this is the time when you practice/play your sport. For military people and first responders, I recommend a long run/fast hike at least twice a month. I like to alternate a weight vest hump with a long slow run without the vest. There is something about running/hiking for an extended time that conditions and toughens your body (and mind) in a way that nothing else can. You don't have to go fast—just shoot for at least five miles (for the run) within your hour. You could run and walk, or just walk, but if you walk put some effort into it and make it real PT. Obviously, if you want to train for running road races or even a marathon, you'll be doing a lot more running. I'm talking here just about general conditioning.

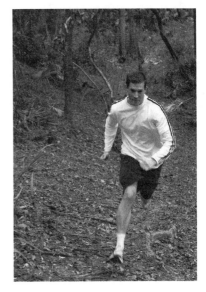

While I'm on the subject of running, get the best shoes you can afford. I ran for years like a dummy in high-top leather basketball sneakers (and two pair of tube socks) and I still like to run in boots as much as possible. However, the long-term benefits of wearing high-quality, well-fitted running shoes cannot be overstated. Figure out your foot and stride type and get the right type of shoe—it can make a huge difference in your running and in how well your body holds up to running. Also don't be cheap and wear them till they have holes in them. I go through a pair of running shoes every two to three months. Your feet and knees will let you know when they're worn out. In a pinch you can buy a set of gel inserts to extend the life of your running shoes a few weeks if you're in a place where no good running shoes are available.

With Support PT, for the most part you have the flexibility to do what you like to do. But remember, you need to pick something that is really PT. Playing softball while drinking beer in the dugout (been there, done that) is not what I'm talking about here. The same goes for touch football. I also don't include golf on this list as, to me, it's not really exercise, not the kind to get you in real shape. Nothing against golf but I've seen some very overweight people herding together on the golf course; that alone should tell you something.

Cycling and Swimming
A few years back I really got into triathlons. I spent a lot of time on a bike and in the pool training for these events. The cycling part took some education. I was lucky there because an officer I worked for had been racing bikes for years. He got me up to speed on the basic ins and outs of cycling, which, if you've never done it seriously, is very extensive. The bikes, the gear, the training, etc.—it can be a lot to get your head around without help. I'm not talking about getting a mountain bike from Wal-Mart and pedaling around the block. Cycling is a world unto itself, and it's much harder than it looks.

The more I got into that part of triathlon racing, the more respect I had for guys like Lance Armstrong. Road racing is a very tough sport at even the lowest levels. What he has done makes him seem superhuman to me. The training can be brutal if you really work at it. The sickest (puking sick) I ever got from exercise-induced exhaustion was during one of our infamous Wednesday-night bike sprint workouts. It can be some serious PT, but if you get yourself a good bike, set it up right, and get with someone in the know, you'll mostly figure it out.

That is not the case with swimming, however. I first got interested in this when I was stationed in upstate New York on recruiting duty. Now, recruiting duty is a story in itself, but to make a long story short, I had survived the

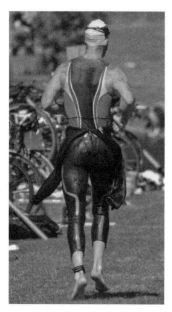

actual recruiting part for three years, and then extended (don't ask why) my tour to come up to be the operations chief at the head shed. This was almost a normal job compared to being a canvassing recruiter. Your hours are still long, but it's pretty normal comparatively.

My executive officer (XO) and operations officer (OpsO) were big into PT like myself so we started doing different races together on the weekends. We had kind of a local Marine Corps team, and we did these events to highlight the Marine Corps to help the local recruiting effort, public relations–type stuff. We did dual-a-tons (where you bike and run) and 5 and 10k runs. We even did a stair-climbing race up the Corning Tower in Albany. We actual did pretty well in a few of them, and it was a good way to stay in shape. The families would come and watch us. It was a fun thing all around and helped take the edge off the pressures of recruiting duty.

When the weather started to warm up, we heard about a race up at Saratoga Lake, by the famous horseracing track. It was a triathlon, and you could do it as a team. I think it was a mile swim, a 50-mile bike ride, and a 10k run. The XO was the best runner and the OpsO was the big bike guy, so that left yours truly with the mile swim. No biggie, I thought. The race was about a month away so I went down to the local community center and started swimming. I had never swum in a race before in my life, but I was in great running shape and I was a good swimmer (or at least I thought so); I'd been able to swim all my life. I went down there early in the morning a couple of times a week and swam. No technique, just splashing back and forth. After a few weeks, I felt I was ready to race.

The day of the race was cool and overcast, and the water looked pretty rough. I would say it was about 60 degrees and windy, but the water was warm enough and I had borrowed a high-speed wet suit from a friend so I thought no big deal. We all signed in and got our stuff together. At some point all the swimmers were called to the water's edge to get our pre-race brief. There were about 300 of us crowded on that little beach.

A guy on a bull horn said, "See that big orange float out there?"

I strained my eyes to see something that looked like an orange basketball way out in the middle of the lake. (It was actually a half mile away).

The guy continued, "That is your turn-around marker. Swim around the marker and then back to the beach for the swim portion of this race. If you're doing this in a team, you must be out of the water before you hand it off."

Each team had to carry a belt and hand it off to each member to carry, start to finish. I had ours around my waist. I was ready.

As I looked around, some of the people who were lined up to do this looked like swimmers, but not that many, however. Most looked of average build. There were also many younger kids and, surprisingly, quite a few older folks. I wondered if I should get to the front so I wouldn't have to go around all these people. I decided instead just to go to the outside of the pack to avoid the initial crush as everyone hit the water.

The horn went off and, like a pack of walruses being chased by a polar bear, we hit the surf. After about a half hour of furious splashing, I was exhausted and stopped swimming to rest. Like a German U-boat scanning for allied ships, I popped my head up to check things out. To my surprise (and horror), I was only about halfway to the float. I looked back toward shore and the people on the beach looked like dots. (Distance over water is hard to figure.) But the worst thing was that of about 300 people swimming, I was in about 299th place, maybe last. Huh? And I was pretty tired already.

My pride didn't let me turn back so I started doggie-paddling my way forward as fast as I could. Fast is a relative term here, and any five-year-old wearing water wings could've passed me. Man, it was slow going. That stupid belt around my waist felt like lead. I looked more like a manatee grubbing for kelp than somebody in a swimming race.

After a short while, I met the other swimmers coming back the other way. They were stroking along like a pod of dolphins. It was all I could do to just get out of their way. About the time I was wishing that a giant catfish would just swallow me and get this torture over with, I got to the turn-around point. To my surprise, the "little" orange float was about 6 to 8 feet high and I could barely see the shore from there. It felt like I had just abandoned the *Titanic*. But reaching the turn-around point did perk me up a little so I turned and paddled for home. This went on for what seemed like hours. About halfway back, I became aware of a swimmer off to the right of me. I could see it was a woman because of her bathing cap but I couldn't tell anything more. She was swimming with way better style than me, but not really going any faster.

At this point I was determined at least not to be the last one out of the water, so I pushed myself as hard as I could go. Which was about the speed of a glacier moving down a mountain. Just before I felt like I was going to drown, my feet felt the bottom. The beach actually ran quite a ways out in the water.

"Thank Christ," I thought as I went to stand up. However, I was so spent my legs wouldn't support me and I fell over backwards. The shore was still at least 100 yards away. Out to my right I caught a glimpse of the other swimmer getting to her feet. To my shock it was a very old lady. When I say old, I mean old. White as a ghost and wrinkled like a prune. I was horrified that a Miss America contestant from the 1937 pageant was going to beat me out of the water.

She got right up and started for land. Now I had to beat this woman or I would never live it down. I managed to haul myself up and tried to run, but all I could do was walk. I staggered like a drunk at Mardi Gras. She seemed to be just casually walking. I could hear the crowd at the beach cheering us on. It became a death match between me and the lady from *Murder, She Wrote*. Finally we got to the water's edge and, looking out of the corner of my eye, I knew it was going to be close. I could see the OpsO in his bike gear waiting for me to hand him the belt. My wife and kids were yelling for me to hurry up. With all the strength I could gather I tore the belt from my waist and lunged forward to hand it off. With that I hit the sand face first, completely spent. Spitting the sand from my mouth, I looked up to see if the OpsO had made it to his bike yet, but to my horror all I saw was the droopy ass of an 80-year-old woman running up the beach (from ground level, no less). If there were a sharp sea shell anywhere near me, I would've gouged my eyes out. She had beaten me!

I relate this embarrassing story to help make a point. If you don't know how to swim (and I mean swim correctly, not just tread water), it won't make any difference how fast you can run or ride a bike. You'll damn near drown like I did. It's a whole different thing. If you have any desire to do a triathlon, you need to get some lessons. Which is what I did after that, and it made a huge difference. I started taking swimming lessons from an old Russian guy at the Jewish community center in town.

The first day, as a bunch of new students were standing at the pool's edge, he said to me, "You there, tough guy, jump in water, swim to end, and come back fast, now go!"

"Yes, sir," I shouted from years of Marine reflex, and dove right in. I tried to do my best impression of a swimmer and went as fast as I could.

I got back (exhausted like always) and he reached down and took my pulse at my neck. He said, "You, you very strong man, no can swim." He was right.

I learned a lot from him, too much to relate to you here. It's enough to say that swimming is a real skill, not just a test of conditioning. Books don't really help much here, either. You need a coach to actually take you through the proper strokes, adjust your technique, and design the right workouts. It's very similar to boxing in this regard.

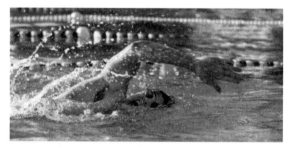

I will pass on one simple swimming workout for you to do, if you don't really care about swimming speed or technique. It's a simple workout to build pure endurance, as simple and effective as it gets. You don't even need goggles (I always wear a diving mask when swimming. I never could get used to those little goggles. They make me feel like the Creature from the Black Lagoon.) Just go to any pool where you can swim laps. All you do here is swim back and forth under water. You can use fins if you want. Just come up when you need a breath, then go back down and keep going. It isn't much for developing swim speed but it will develop some serious lung power as you do all your swimming while holding your breath. Try to get in as many laps as you can in an hour. It's my favorite swim workout, both effective and a true no-brainer. Swimming also will give your joints a break from running and cycling. It's a great Support workout if you have a pool you can use. I know what you're thinking: NO, drinking beer in a jacuzzi doesn't count as swimming.

CHAPTER 6

ACTIVE REST

Active rest? Sounds like a play on words, and it is in a way. However, I put these words together to try and describe something in the right way. We all know that along with hard exercise you must get enough rest to recuperate both mentally and physically. If you don't, you'll overtrain, burn out, or, even worse, get injured. We need adequate sleep and a good diet to start, but we also need to relax mentally. So when you think of rest, the first thing that may come to mind is someone just hanging out, sitting on the beach or in a soft chair mesmerized by the idiot box or a laptop. That type of rest is sometimes good, but a better type of rest is something that is also easy and laidback, but includes some actual movement of your body.

I first heard of this technique many years ago. When I was competing in Olympic lifting, I trained at a friend's house. His father was at one time a nationally ranked Olympic-style power lifter. He had a nice home gym and a basement full of trophies he had won over the years. Also down there was a big pile of old musty muscle magazines. After we worked out we would sit around and shoot the breeze with his father (his father also worked at the local bakery and always had a ton of cookies and other nasty baked goods for us to grub on) and read those old magazines. Most were from the '60s and '70s, motivating old stuff.

Anyhow, I remember one article about the Soviet Olympic weightlifting team (don't ask me how I remember all this stuff, it just sticks in my head). Back in those days the Soviets were the powerhouse in Olympic-style weightlifting. This article mentioned that the team stayed "active" during their off time from training with things like light jogging, recreational sports, and lots of walking. The Soviet theory was that this kept the guys loose (mentally and physically) and made it easier to manage their body weight (rather than just sitting around). My friend's father told us this was something they always used when training for a lifting meet. I always thought this made sense, and found it to be true for me and for others. I've been doing it and recommending it ever since.

I'm always much less sore the day after a hard run or PT if I go for at least a walk or do something other than sit around later that same day. It's also important from an attitude standpoint.

Here are some common examples of active rest:

- Yard/house work
- Vehicle maintenance (washing the car, etc.)
- Golfing
- Walking
- Light bike riding (like around the neighborhood)
- Throwing horseshoes, shooting baskets
- Motorcycle riding (road)
- Most hunting and fishing

There are many other things that fit in this category. An important thing to remember with this is while active rest on its own will not (in most cases) get you into any real condition, it will burn some calories, which can

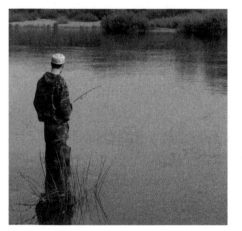

make a big difference in managing your weight. If you've traveled overseas, you'll note that you see much fewer overweight people; in some countries you'd be hard-pressed to find anyone overweight. It's not because they all eat a perfect diet or exercise 24/7. It's because they're much more active than Americans in their everyday lives, meaning they walk and ride bikes everywhere. However, don't confuse the fact that an activity that makes you tired is real PT. Fishing on the ocean all day in the hot sun will tire you out, but it's not exercise.

This stuff is very important for your attitude. To me, there's nothing better than riding my Harley on a nice day. Almost nothing else will relax me or recharge my batteries better, but I know it's not exercise. I recommend that you consciously include active rest into your overall fitness plan every day, especially doing as much as you can out of doors. There is something about being outside in the fresh air that will rejuvenate you much better than anything you can do inside, especially if your job keeps you cooped up all day. Turn off the TV or the computer, get off your rear and go wash the car, walk the dog, or play catch with your kids. Especially after you eat dinner.

MAKING IT WORK

CHAPTER 7

PLANNING

They (meaning the 50-pound brains) say that in combat, tactics win battles, but logistics win wars. In a nutshell, it'll be the planning and the better supply chain that will probably determine the outcome, not the brilliant flanking maneuvers. Those who can get to the right place the fastest, with the most people and all their stuff, will win. The same goes for PT and eating right. Planning is important when it comes to PT.

So far we've been talking about the tactics of getting you in shape, how to train and eat. Now we need to talk the logistics of when, where, and how to make training part of YOUR life, not the other way around.

One of the first (and most important) things that you have to consider is when to PT. The overall answer is simple but needs to be really thought through to make it work for you long term. As you can probably guess by now, I'm not interested in short-term fixes; what I'm looking for are lasting, long-term results. The right habits and the right mindset are key here, so you need to think this through.

Over the years, I've done PT at every possible time in a 24-hour day. Day, night, midnight, "0 dark 30," you name it. That's because during my time in the Marines, I worked all different shifts, and many of these places had gyms, or at least a safe place to PT 24/7. So what's the best time to work out? The best time is the time that you find is the best for you, your schedule, your energy level, etc. That may sound too simple or vague, but that's the right answer. You really have to figure it out for yourself. However, I'll give you some important things to consider.

Personally, I think the best time to PT is when you first wake up, whenever that is. When I worked "nights," that was about noon. When I worked "mids," that was around 7 p.m. When I was a recruiter, that was 6 a.m. When I was in Iraq, that was 5 a.m. When I was running the Ordnance school house in Pensacola, we started PT at 04. My point here is that getting up early and starting your day with a PT is one of the absolute best things you can do for yourself, on many levels.

For one thing, once you get used to it (in about a week or so), your energy level will be at its highest. This is especially true for first responders or anyone who has a very physical job. I know how hard it is to PT after a full day of construction work or working on the flight deck of a Navy ship in the hot sun. You can do it, but it can be very tough to do long term. I know from my own experience in the construction business that during the summer months, you'll almost always work till dark. Contractors (especially up north) will try to get all the work in they can during the warmer months, using the longer daylight times. With that, you're going to want to take advantage of this and work all the overtime you can get. That's what I did. So I know that trying to do any PT after 10 to 12 hours of physical work in the hot summer months is tough going.

However, maybe the best thing about exercising first thing is that it's the time that will be less influenced by events later in your day. Simply put, you get up early and get it over with. So no matter what comes up (and trust me, things will always come up), your PT is in the bank. There are other benefits, such as gyms are less crowded and, if you decide to run down your street, there's little traffic to worry about. From another angle, it's a great attitude booster. Some of you reading this will think I'm a mental patient for saying this, but for me there's just something about starting a run in the dark and finishing it as the sun rises (just remember to always wear reflective clothing when running in anything other than broad daylight). It starts your day on a positive note like nothing else can. It's my all-time favorite time to train, but I realize this isn't everyone's cup of tea. Some people just don't like to get up early, let alone exercise right away. So they have to come up with a better time. My general rule is the earlier the better, so here are the three most common times to train after first thing in the morning: at lunch, right after work (before dinner), after dinner. I've done all of these and can offer insight on them.

Lunch-hour PT can be good—it's a great way to break up your work day and refreshes you for the afternoon. Of course, this depends on your job and, more specifically, your working hours. Many people reading this only get a half hour for lunch, or they work at a place (construction site, assembly line, restaurant, retail shop) where this is simply not practical. However, many large companies have located gyms within their company spaces and offer longer lunch breaks to workers who choose to exercise during lunch (this helps with their insurance costs). If they offer this at your work, you should take full advantage of it. Most firehouses and police departments have a gym of some type set up, and the personnel can PT in between calls.

There are a few pros and cons to doing PT right after work, before dinner. One of the pros is that you're done with work, and it's a great way to work off the stress of the day before you go home. If you're forced or choose to exercise at this time, I strongly suggest that you PT before you go home. I know from experience that (unless you're single) once you step in the door, you'll have a hard time getting to PT. Something will come up. (Trust me. I've been through this.) The kids will jump on you, your spouse will have something for you to do, or the smell of dinner will distract you. This all makes it too easy to skip your training. Also, there are always social considerations. Remember what I said about "support for your life, not your life"? There will be times, especially on Thursday or Friday nights, when you want to do something right after work, maybe have a few beers with coworkers, meet your family for a dinner out, or watch your kid's basketball game. You're going to gaff off your PT when this happens. And you know what? You should. Your family should always take priority in that kind of standoff. My point is that you need to set up your routine in such a way to minimize these kinds of choices.

The last time to work out (and the worst, in my opinion) is at night after dinner. This is a bad long-term choice all the way around. First, you'll be tired, both from a day of work and your dinner. You'll feel groggy and sleepy, and you won't have much energy for PT. Plus, if you do manage to get one in, you'll have trouble sleeping because exercise wakes you up and makes it hard to relax/sleep for a few hours. If you choose to PT at this time, you'll have a very hard time maintaining this schedule. You'd be much better off getting up at 4 a.m. to exercise. In other words, I highly recommend that you don't make this your exercise time if you can in any way help it. But if you're a night owl, this may be the best for you. In the end, the most important thing is that you set up a workout time that will work for you long term.

Speaking of long term, I laid out a sample month-long schedule in Appendix E to help you get started. Feel free to use it or make up your own.

PT while Traveling or on Vacation

When you're traveling for business or on vacation, the last thing you'll probably want to think about is PT. However, in my experience these are two of the most important times to PT, *especially* if you travel a lot.

Let's start with business travel. I've logged thousands of miles traveling around this country for deployments, conferences, and schools. You name the place, I've probably been there. I've slept in so many different places in my life that I sometimes wake up and for a few seconds don't know where I am. All the deployments, trips, motels, and barracks rooms all start to look alike after a while. So when it comes to PT on the fly, I speak from experience.

The key to making this work is simple planning. On the day of travel, you should try to (if at all possible) book your flight for 9 a.m. or even later. Why? So you can get in some PT before you go to the airport or start driving. This practice has many benefits, one being that you'll miss the big morning crowd at the airport or the local rush hour as everyone else tries to travel early for business. I used to do the same thing,

Packing for PT on the Go

With most airlines charging you extra for heavy and/or extra luggage nowadays, carrying PT clothes is not a worry. A pair of running shoes and a couple of sets of PT clothes don't weigh squat. Forget about bringing water dumbbells, push-up handles, or other so-called portable PT stuff—it's really just junk and not worth the money or effort to haul around. Also, I don't really think much of those in-room workout routines that you hear about. Other than maybe doing some push-ups, abs, and stretching, you're much better off actually finding a gym than wasting your time.

And while you're at it, pack yourself a good lunch to eat while you're traveling. Airport food makes me want to jump off a roof. It's for the most part expensive, greasy garbage. If you want to feel really lousy after a long plane trip, load up on bad airport coffee and fast food as you fly coast to coast (especially east to west). I know people who do this all the time, and then they wonder why they're exhausted and feel sick when they get to where they're going. Make a couple of good sandwiches and take some fruit. If you need some incentive, just take a look around at all of the sumo wrestlers in line at the airport food court. If that doesn't scare you, throw away this book and head to McDonald's.

and unless you have to be at a meeting that day or something, it's really a dumb idea. I used to get to where I was going so early, I couldn't even check into my room for a few hours. Then what? Some will say that they have office work to do that day and need to be there early, but if you're giving a brief or a presentation, shouldn't you have it mostly done before you get on the road? When traveling, like always, things come up. Your flight may get delayed, your luggage might get lost. That's why I recommend that you always try to get some PT in prior to starting travel whenever possible.

Another big benefit of getting in some PT before you travel is that it'll take the edge off, both physically and mentally. We all know how airports are nowadays, and I feel better all around when I PT first. I can handle the waiting around and the longer flights better when I'm a little drowsy from PT. It's when you're wide awake and keyed up that you'll have trouble getting comfortable while traveling. You may even be able to relax enough to catch some shut-eye.

If you have to travel early, plan on getting some PT in when you get there. When you make your hotel reservation, ask about their facilities. Nowadays most places have something, whether a treadmill, a pool, or a rowing machine. Those that don't have in-house gyms may give out free passes to a local gym in the area. If that's the case, you can check out that gym online, or call them to get their hours and what they have available. Again, a little planning goes a long way. This can help you unwind after the trip.

After you arrive at your hotel and get situated, you should keep to your normal routine as best as you can. If there's no gym around, take a drive and find a park or a school where you can PT. There's always one or the other nearby. If you're in a place that has a couple of floors, you could run or walk the stairs. I've done this more than once, especially in bad weather. Doing your normal training will keep your mind sharp for whatever business you're doing, and it'll help you sleep better. Make PT part of your trip and plan for it like any other part.

Vacation travel is basically the same planning-wise, but there are a few differences. While you don't have the worry of work over your head, there are things you want to do. You've probably spent a bunch of money to go someplace and you don't want to waste your time. The point is to have fun and relax. So when it comes to vacations, the bottom line is to just get up in the morning and PT every day before you move on to vacation stuff. It's been my experience that you can forget about trying to do anything later in the day. Trust me when I tell you that you'll enjoy your vacation more during and after you get home if you PT at least a little while you're there. It's not that hard, so stop whining and get up and go. We're talking at the most an hour, remember? Then you come back awake and ready to do whatever. Keep in mind that you're going to eat and drink more while on vacation. Keeping up your PT will head off that weight gain that many put on during vacations.

When my kids were little, I'd get up early to train while my wife slept in. When I got back, she'd go and do her PT. By the time the kids got up, we were both done and having coffee, ready to deal with the nightmare of a day with the kids at a theme park. Even Disney has some decent gyms in their hotels, and trust me when I tell you that I never found a crowded one. Mindset and planning are the keys here. If you decide that you're just not going to do any PT while on vacation, be prepared for the weight gain and the battle to get back into shape when you return. A week off can take a month of hard work to get back up to speed. It's not that hard and you'll have a better travel/vacation experience if you do it.

CHAPTER 8

CHOW

If you go by what you see and hear, how to eat right must be the most confusing piece of the staying-in-shape riddle. Just turn on the TV and every other commercial is about food, diets, or weight loss. It's a mental overload if you try and figure out what's true and what's not. If you ask me, 99 percent of it is just media hype—one day this food is bad for you, the next month the same stuff is good for you? The human body hasn't really changed much in thousands of years, but a new diet or weight loss product that came out last week is now the only right way to eat? Please, I don't buy it.

While I think learning how to PT correctly is more complicated than learning the correct way to eat, in the end I think eating right (or wrong) has more influence on your overall health than exercise. Plus I think it's harder to develop good eating habits than exercise habits. I once heard an experienced body builder say the hardest workouts he ever did were with a "knife and fork." I think that anyone who has tried to watch what they eat can relate to that statement.

My thinking with PT has always been to do what's effective and make it fit into your life. I feel exactly the same way about eating. When it comes to eating right, I have my own ideas, based on actual experience, study, and observation. What I mean when I say "eating right" is simply eating for maximum energy, great long-term health, weight management, AND a positive experience. All are important, including the last one. Enjoying good food, especially with friends and family, is one of life's greatest pleasures, one that I've always enjoyed and plan to enjoy for the rest of my life.

I think the single biggest problem that most people have with eating is that they misunderstand, and for some reason mistrust, the basic, tired, and true principles. So instead of following a common-sense direction, they'll try any crazy thing that comes up. In other words, the thinking is screwed up. I've seen many people who are great leaders, very successful and intelligent, try to lose weight on the silliest diets you can think of. The whole concept of trying to eat right seems to make people crazy. I'm not a nutritionist (but I've received guidance from some really good ones) and guess what? I don't need to be, and neither do you to get this mostly right. A great place to start is the USDA website (www.mypyramid.gov), which has lots of good, all-around eating guides.

Everybody is different. What people eat, and the effects of that eating, can vary greatly from person to person. They can vary so greatly it's foolish for anyone to think that what works for one person will definitely work for another. That's why the basic tried and true guidelines are really the only way to go. From here you can adjust for your own goals, activity level, taste, and metabolism. Here's a good example of what I'm talking about.

A few years back, a Marine who was a real body builder worked for me. He wasn't like most people who lift some weights and call themselves body builders. This guy was the real deal. He actually won the Mr. Pensacola title when we were there. He was huge, very strong and ripped, with very little body fat. When he was training for a contest, he'd come into my office every morning and eat two to three nasty, fat-filled vending machine honey buns, dipping them in a big jar of peanut butter. He did this every day right up to the contest. He also constantly ate fast food. I was dumbfounded by his diet as this went against everything that I'd ever read or heard about body-building diets, especially right before a contest. When I questioned him about this, his answer was that he just needed calories, almost any calories, to get in contest shape. It worked for him, as the night of the contest he was about 220 pounds of pure muscle.

The take-away lesson from this is that if the average person ate that way, they'd be pure blubber. His superior genetics and two hours a day spent lifting weights seemed to just convert everything into muscle. (It's important to note that even though he looked great, eating that poor diet at some point would become unhealthy, especially in regards to heart health.) On the other end, I've seen overweight people who actually ate pretty well but had a very hard time managing their weight. Some people may have metabolic disorders or other health issues that need to be addressed by a doctor. In any case, I've seen many examples of this variable between people. So in my opinion, trying to set up a detailed eating plan that will work for everyone is not realistic. I also think that the part of the country/world that you're from has a big influence on your eating habits. So my goal here is to give you some tried and true (simple) guidance to help keep your weight under control, without killing yourself.

The Basics

Here are a few general rules of thumb to healthy eating and weight control.

Eat real food, food from the earth. Fresh fruits and vegetables, whole grains, lean meats, and low-fat dairy are always a good start. Avoid fast food and other processed junk. You don't really need all the expensive organic stuff to be healthy, either, although there's no doubt that organic food is better for you overall and if you can afford to, it would be the way to go. Organic produce has more nutrients, and fewer chemicals were used in their growth and/or processing. Having said all that, many organic foods are more expensive and not always available where you live. As they become more popular, the prices will come down and they'll become more accessible. I do most of my food shopping at the base commissary as I'm retired military, but when that isn't practical, I go right to Wal-Mart. I have no problem with it as their food is good and priced right. Plus, in recent years they've added many organic items throughout their stores. I also highly recommend that you go to local farmer's markets to get fresh fruit and vegetables. Besides getting some great food, you're supporting your local farmers and merchants.

Here's a practical example of what I'm recommending. I've been involved with boxing in one way or another for almost all my adult life. Professional fighters are as physically fit as anyone in the world, and unlike athletes in many high-energy sports (marathon running, football, cycling, etc.), they have to effectively manage their weight to fall within specific weight classes. So you know they have to closely watch what they eat to be able to perform at their best and still make weight.

As a big fan of boxing history, I've read the biography of almost every famous fighter out there. In every single case, when former champions talk about their training routine (from over 100 years ago to the present day) and specifically their training diet, they all ate the same things: simple, wholesome, nutritious food. Nothing fancy, just the basics, and they didn't pig out. This common-sense approach worked for Rocky Marciano, Joe Louis, Muhammad Ali, Roy Jones, Jr., and all the other great fighters, and it'll work for you, too. Keep it basic and simple.

Drink plenty of water—not soda or sports drinks. Plain, pure water is the best. Your body cannot function properly when it's dehydrated; even being slightly dehydrated can cause problems. Get in the habit of always keeping some water around. In 1991 during Operation Desert Storm, I worked on the flight deck of a Navy ship loading heavy ordnance onto Harrier jump jets. The temperature was oftentimes over 120 degrees. Plus we had to wear all our protective gear and work around hot aircraft exhaust. About a dozen of us hand-loaded over

250 tons of ordnance during the three-day ground war. We all drank gallons of water (just water) a day to keep from getting heat exhaustion. We didn't have a single heat casualty or real injury of any type, and that was only because we were trained for it and kept drinking water. If you're a firefighter wearing heavy gear, fighting a fire in summer heat could dehydrate you and cause you to pass out and become a casualty yourself if you don't constantly drink water.

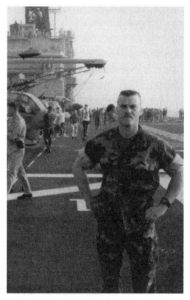

Author Paul Roarke on the flight deck of a Navy ship.

Many sports drinks aren't much better than soda if you read the labels, but I do like regular old-school green Gatorade (it also has an advantage over water as it helps replenish electrolytes). When it's hot and I'm sweating heavily and working hard, it's a great drink. It's not too sweet, and I was once told by a Navy flight surgeon that cold Gatorade cut 50/50 with water will absorb right into your system and won't upset your stomach. The best way to do that is to just mix it with lots of ice (if you have it). As a rule, reach for a water bottle, not a soda can.

Three balanced meals a day are enough. I often see/hear people on the five-to-six-meals-a-day eating plans (you know, the ones where you eat a small meal every two hours or so) trying to lose weight. I'm not saying that can't work, I understand the concept, and it will work if followed to the letter. I just don't think it's practical for most working people. Now, I realize that this goes against all the experts out there. Yeah, well, so what? I go with what I KNOW works. If everybody was able to do what the "experts" recommend, there wouldn't be so many overweight people around. *It's not enough that you say you know what works, you have to be able to do it.*

For me, and I think for most people, it's just too much hassle getting all these little meals together, then having to stop and eat all the time. I'm not a baby, you're not, either, and we don't need to be fed every two hours like one. We all have better things to do than worry about when our next feeding is. I also think your body needs a rest in between meals. If you get really hungry in between, grab a small snack like a piece of fruit. Remember what I said at the start of this book. PT and eating are support for YOUR life, not the other way around. My general rule is to not eat between meals, other than maybe some fruit or a handful of raw nuts. No, this doesn't cause me to eat like an escaped convict when I do eat my meals. In fact, by not eating in between, I feel full more quickly when I do eat. I even have a special secret name for this method: eating like an adult. Try it.

Eat a large variety of good foods. No single food has everything you need in it to keep you healthy. A good rule of thumb is to try to eat at least 15 different foods a day. Have a little bit of everything. Another way to look at it is to get as many different-colored foods as you can. Mixing things up will also make you feel more satisfied and less likely to overeat. Try new foods; it's good for you mentally as well as physically. Just don't get too crazy. In Thailand, I ate a fried scorpion on a bet. I didn't know I was supposed to break off the stinger beforehand (hey, it was my first) and he managed to sting my lower lip on the way down. My lip swelled up like an inner tube, and I was in a semiconscious state for about two days. I don't remember much about those two days, but I do remember that scorpion—it was buttcrack nasty. Eat a little of everything, but make sure it's dead first.

Eat till you're full then stop. This is a simple concept but not easy for most people to do. If you can't go by the feeling of being full, you'll have to use another one of your senses, namely your eyesight. I'll assume you can see your plate (not a tray or a platter, either, Jethro—a normal-sized dinner plate). A full plate of anything at one sitting is plenty. Use your eyeballs to determine the proper portion of something. A potato should be about the size of a hard ball, not a football. You don't need a 16-ounce steak; 8 ounces of high-quality meat is more than plenty for one meal. If you're eating pasta, rice, or a casserole, one good scoop is enough. Most people eat too fast, so slow down. It takes some time for your brain to realize you've had enough. Relax and enjoy your food. Try putting your fork down between bites. Think about it: When you're really hungry, the best part of a meal is the first few bites, not the part where you keep cramming it in until you're stuffed like a deer tick. Remember: Enough is as good as a feast.

Enjoy some favorite foods once in a while. Let's face it: The fattening foods are the ones that taste great (I personally like burgers, barbecue, hot wings, pizza, etc.). Don't give them up. Just have them once in a while, and you'll enjoy them more as a treat. It's not special if you do it everyday; try once a week.

Here's what I do: Once a week I'll have a "blowout" meal, but not a full blowout day, like some fitness guides will recommend. A full day of pigging out is foolish and unhealthy. A "blowout" meal means you can have whatever you want, and I mean anything (steak, fried chicken, baked potato with sour cream, burgers, pizza), including dessert (pie and ice cream).

It sounds good, doesn't it? But first you have to earn it. Earn a blowout meal by first eating right the majority of the time (a good rule of thumb is the 80/20 rule, meaning that you eat right 80 percent of the time and stray no more than 20 percent) and putting in a hard PT session before you eat it. In my mind, a long run or bike ride is the best way to do this. Then follow the "Rule of One": ONE full plate and ONE dessert. That's it. ONE means ONE. UNO. No seconds, and you have to eat it all at one setting. No saving dessert for later. One full heaping plate of great food—a big meal with a nice dessert. When you're done, you'll feel fat, dumb, and happy. You can make this a regular thing, like a Sunday brunch or Saturday cookout. But once a week only, one meal only, and one helping only. Just make sure you earn it first.

High-Performance Eating

On any given morning at military bases, hundreds of Marines, soldiers, sailors, and airmen undergo command PT before heading to work for the day. This routine is considered an important component of military readiness. Similarly, many civilians commonly start their workouts without eating. If you're one of these people, you may want to consider the importance of eating before getting down to business.

The importance of eating before exercise, better known in the sports nutrition community as "frontloading," is important for topping off carbohydrate stores in the muscles and providing energy to exert maximum effort during strenuous exercise sessions. Breaking the overnight fast with a well-balanced breakfast consisting of a serving of whole-grain cereal (such as steel cut oats), a serving of low-fat dairy, and a piece of fruit will increase the basal metabolic rate (BMR). This is an important factor in maintaining a healthy body weight because, in simple terms, eating before exercise "stokes your internal fire," increasing the rate at which calories are burned. This practice will also help prevent binging on less nutrient-rich snacks later in the day. Re-fueling during exercise is not necessary if workouts are less than an hour. For long bouts of exercise (over an hour), it's recommended that approximately 1 gram of carbohydrate per minute is consumed during these extended evolutions. Many endurance athletes replenish themselves with beverages containing both carbohydrates and important electrolytes such as sodium and potassium. These drinks not only provide important nutrients, but also fluids.

Another important consideration over the past few years involves nutrition and, in particular, nutrition recovery. According to many researchers studying sports nutrition, what is eaten, especially immediately after PT, plays a key component to performance success. Without food in the tank, the engine is at a disadvantage when it comes to energy sustainment and next-day all-out PT effort. The human engine has a recovery window of about 30–45 minutes post-exercise that requires a refueling strategy consisting of a mixed meal of protein and carbohydrate. Foods high in carbohydrate will enable a fuel injection of sugar to enter muscles and store what is needed for the next day's requirement of primary energy, while protein provides the amino acids required to keep a positive protein balance to prevent catabolism or muscle breakdown. A recovery meal using real food instead of dietary supplements gives the "weapon's platform" (human body) more bang for its buck in nutrients. Real food is also leaner in the long run when it comes to the pocketbook. Examples of good recovery fuel include a cup of low-fat chocolate milk, a whole-grain bagel with natural peanut butter, or half a turkey sandwich. Men, in particular, are notorious for waiting at the end of the day to eat because of the high operational tempo of the work day or mission. Navy SEAL food logs indicate that over 60% of calories are consumed after 18:00. This habit is not only detrimental to performance, but a health nightmare—one common result is weight gain, particularly in the belly, which may result in comorbidities such as hyperlipidemia, hypertension, and diabetes. By eating more calories during the first half of the waking hours and remembering to re-fuel immediately after exercise, health sustainability and longevity will guarantee long-term high performance and lower the likelihood of injury.

Eat at the house. Buy good fresh food and cook it yourself. Pack your own lunch. Try to not eat out more than once a week. If you keep track, you'll find most people eat out much more than they realize. It's also a waste of money. When you're traveling, that's a different story, but it's still better if you buy good food and eat in your room for most of your meals, especially if you can get a room with a kitchenette, or at least a microwave and small fridge. Fresh home-cooked meals have always been the best, and always will be. On an economic note, when you choose to eat out, go to a local place instead of one of the big chain restaurants. Not only will they have the fresher, healthier food, you'll be supporting your local economy, which is always important.

Lastly, don't fall for it. This means stop trying every new diet that comes out. Again, the human body hasn't really changed in thousands of years, so what makes you think that a new diet that came out last week is the way to go? It's silly. The basics are the key. Why? Because they work.

Losing Weight

In the last section I gave you some general tips on eating. These general guidelines are really all you need to maintain your weight and feel and perform at your best. If you're overweight, stick with my PT program and use common sense when eating—you'll get down to your natural weight. It may take some time, but it'll happen.

Before we go any further into weight loss, we need to talk about what that means, "natural weight." As you know, people are different and come in all shapes and sizes. Some are naturally thin, some are stocky. They also have different metabolisms and different levels of activity. All of these things influence a person's weight. Age also has some influence on this, but not as much as you'd think.

As always, you have to get your thinking right first, because every overweight person out there has a weight in their head or written down somewhere as a goal. I think that goals are great, as long as they're developed using your half a brain and not some picture in a fitness magazine or some nonsense you saw on a TV infomercial. So first off, stop comparing yourself to professional fitness models and athletes.

I've seen many charts and studies about the ideal body weight for any given height, build, and age. I actually think many of those charts are a pretty good standard to go by. While I know some will not agree with me, they give you a good general idea to work from, or your job may have its own (insurance companies) standards that you have to meet. From my own observations and experience, this is something you really have to figure out for yourself. I'll say that I think being leaner/lighter is better overall for not only appearance, but for performance and overall health.

Let me illustrate this in a simple way. In the wild you have lions and you have leopards. Everybody wants to be the lion, "king of beasts" and all that. Even if you're born smaller, like myself, and are more like a leopard (although, according to my son, I'm more like a badger), you try to turn yourself into a lion. That's not going to happen. I've tried, trust me. I lifted heavy weights, ate huge portions, and took all kinds of supplements (but no steroids). Did I become a lion? No. I was just a sluggish, bloated, and overweight leopard. My weight went as high as 190 pounds, most of it muscle. I was pretty strong and I could run, but I wasn't at my best. I wasn't a kick-ass leopard—I was just a chunky wannabe-lion. After a while (about 20 years, as I'm a slow learner), I figured this out and adjusted my PT and eating habits. Soon I was leopard size (165 pounds) and feeling, looking, and performing much better.

The point here is to get yourself to where you should be, not what someone or something tells you your weight should be. Only you can figure out what the right weight is for you. I would recommend that you go by how you feel and perform first, followed by how you look, and finally by what the scale says. If you're moving well, feel strong (joint problems can be an indication you're carrying too much weight), and aren't carrying any excess fat, you're probably pretty close to where you need to be. You'll know when you get there. The funny thing is that most guys want to be bigger, but with women it's the opposite. They all want to be smaller. Either way you need to find the right balance.

As a simple reference point to start from, try this. Look back to when you thought you were at your best weight. Unless you were overweight or very skinny, this was probably in your early to mid-20s. For example, when I joined the Marine Corps at age 21, I weighed about 150 pounds at 5'7". I was in great shape from daily hard physical work and training as a boxer. As I got older, I continued to PT quite a bit, but my weight slowly went up. I crept up to almost 190 pounds, but normally hovered around 180 pounds. I was in good condition, but I knew I was just too heavy. After changing my thinking, routine, and eating habits, I eventually got to about 165, where I almost instantly felt better. Now, 165 is about 15 pounds over my best, which is a 10 percent increase. So going by my own experience with this, I think that regardless of age, staying within 10 percent of your best weight is a good goal, but in the end you'll have to be honest with yourself when doing this.

To lose weight, you have to do one of two things (or more likely a little of both): increase your activity level, or reduce your food intake. If you follow my program and are also pretty active otherwise, in time your weight will (slowly) stabilize to where it should be. If you follow my program for 30 days and aren't losing the weight you want, you need to adjust your eating, *not your PT*. If you're really using all the EPRS guidance I've laid out and are pushing yourself fairly hard three to five times a week, with plenty of active rest in between, that's all you need. If you try to add another several hours of real exercise, you'll either burn out or injure yourself. Either way you won't be able to maintain it for very long. You could try to add some more active rest, but most likely what you need to do is just tighten up on your eating habits.

I've had many years of experience helping and observing Marines trying to lose weight and keep it off. My general observation from all that is a few basic changes in eating habits, with consistent effort, is all it takes. Here are some simple methods that I know work to lose weight the right way:

Go low fat. This is probably the most effective way to lose weight long term. It's effective for a few reasons. First, it's healthy to reduce fat in your diet, as it's common knowledge that a diet high in saturated fats causes heart disease. Yes, some fats are good, but all fat is very high in calories. So if you eat lower-fat foods, you can still eat a fair amount of good food from a normal-sized menu *and* keep your overall calories down enough to lose weight. Switch to non-fat milk, low-fat cheese, and yogurt. Eat more chicken and fish instead of pork and beef. Avoid fried and other processed foods. High-fat foods are also hard to digest and make you sluggish. Think in terms of eating a "clean" diet. Low-fat foods are like high-octane racing fuel for your body. High-fat foods are more like diesel fuel. Whole milk is like liquefied bacon—read the labels. Look for very low overall fat, meaning less than three grams per serving, and zero grams of saturated and trans-fat.

Drastically reduce or stop your alcohol intake (beer and other alcoholic beverages). They really will pack on the weight. Especially beer. I love beer, but drink a couple of beers a day everyday and you'll soon be a food blister. No easy way to say it: just cut way back on the drinking or you'll stay overweight. It's that simple.

Eat breakfast. There has been study after study done on this: A good breakfast has a big impact on weight loss. It stokes up your metabolism for the day, and it's been proven that people who eat a good breakfast do better at managing their weight. Just make sure you eat something good, like a bowl of low-sugar, high-fiber cereal with some non-fat milk and some fruit. The worst thing for breakfast is the greasy fast-food egg-and-whatever sandwich, or going the doughnut/Danish route. I know many people don't like to eat when they first wake up (I don't), so take your breakfast to work to eat the first chance you get. This is a matter of habit more than anything else.

Drink more water. I covered this in the general guideline section, but I'm bringing it up again as it's important for those who are trying to lose weight. Other drinks like soda, sports drinks, and even fruit juice have a lot of calories, and in many cases excess salt (sodium). They're very concentrated food. A big glass of 100 percent OJ has the calories of about three large oranges in it. Switching to water can make a big difference in helping you lose weight, along with all the other health benefits it brings you.

Don't eat too much at night, and try not to eat at least two hours before you go to bed. After you eat dinner, get in some active rest. If you get really hungry, have non-fat yogurt or even a glass of non-fat milk before bed. I find that a cup of decaf herbal tea helps me sleep and keep me from eating at night. You'll also sleep better without a full meal in your stomach.

Losing weight is more about attitude and consistent effort than anything else. The worst thing you can do to lose weight is to try some new wonder diet or, even worse, rely on diet supplements. Supplements are for the most part a waste of money and, if abused, can be dangerous. I know as I wasted a bunch of money myself over the years, only to figure out that 99 percent of them don't really work. They'll yield short-term results, but nothing long term after your body gets used to them. What are you going to do, take that crap for the rest of your life?

I'll tell you the same thing I used to tell friends when I saw them buying/using expensive supplements. I'd ask, "What if I can show you how to get better results than what you're getting with those products, and it will cost you half as much money?" They always wanted to know how. Here's how it's done: First, take half the money you spend per month on supplements and put that in your pocket. That's your savings. Then give me the other half. Every time I see you I'll tell you how good you look. I'll also tell other people how good you look. I'll tell them you lost weight and look like you're getting in great shape. Sounds funny, but the sad fact is that nine times out of ten, those compliments would be the only real results you'd ever see from all the money you spend on that stuff. I take a good multivitamin every day and recommend the same, but if you're eating well, you don't really need it. It's just insurance, and that can't hurt.

I also recommend avoiding as much of those prepackaged diet foods you see on TV and at the store, the ones with a nice picture on the box that you can sometimes order right to your house. Read the labels: they have tons of preservatives and sodium. What you're paying for is the convenience of just grabbing something in a box or a bag rather than having to buy and cook it. Don't be lazy. It's just a habit to take the time to prepare and eat good, fresh food.

As I stated at the beginning of this chapter, I firmly believe that general guidelines are the best way to eat for maximum performance, staying healthy, and LONG-term weight management. It's because they allow you the flexibility you need to be able to eat right within your normal life schedule. However, I also know that many (if not most) people, especially those who are trying to lose weight, need something tangible to plan around. On page 67 is the exact plan I first used many years ago and still use when I need to drop some weight. It was based on the diet I followed when I was boxing and needed to be able to work a full-time job, box, and keep my

Sample Eating Plan

Calories: *1800* **Protein:** *125 grams* **Carbohydrates:** *250 grams*
Fat: *35 grams (very little saturated fat)* **Fiber:** *40 grams*

BREAKFAST
- Big bowl of low-sugar, low-fat, high-fiber cereal (or oatmeal) with non-fat milk and some fruit (I like Kashi GoLean with blueberries and/or a small banana)
- 1 hard-boiled egg (get the omega-3 eggs)
- Black coffee or tea (no milk and sugar—that's called Girl Scout coffee in the Marine Corps)

MID-MORNING SNACK (if you must)
- Piece of fresh fruit OR a small, non-fat yogurt

LUNCH
- Large bowl of soup (no milk-based soups) with wheat crackers or a big sandwich (turkey, chicken, etc., but not a burger) OR a big tossed salad with some grilled chicken or fish, with light dressing
- Fruit and/or some raw vegetables
- Water or unsweetened iced tea (diet soda if you must drink soda)

MID-AFTERNOON SNACK (if you must)
- Same as in the morning, or maybe a handful of raw nuts or a good trail mix (handful does not mean a bagful)

DINNER
- Large, fresh, tossed salad with light dressing, and/or a cup of clear soup (such as chicken broth; it helps fill you up with almost no calories)
- 6 to 8 oz. of chicken or fish baked, grilled, or broiled (red meat once a week)
- Large serving of vegetables (steamed, boiled, microwaved)
- Reasonable serving (about a cup) of carbs (rice, potato, pasta, or 2 pieces of whole wheat bread)
- Non-fat yogurt or fruit for dessert
- Water or unsweetened iced tea

LATE SNACK (if you must)
- Small bowl of cereal OR a piece of toast with a little peanut butter

weight in a certain weight class. I've recommended this plan to many Marines who were having trouble managing their weight, and they all had success (some had dramatic success) when they followed it. I offer this plan to you because I know it works, and you can add or subtract to it as needed. Having said that, it has a built-in assumption that you're following my PT plan and are fairly active otherwise.

Up till I decided to write this training book, I never had more than a general idea of what the actual calories in my eating plan were, or what the breakdown of protein, carbs, fats, fiber, etc., was. To be honest, I didn't really care because by using my half a brain, my eyes, and the way I felt, I knew it was the right amount of everything to keep me going strong while keeping my weight under control.

However, for instructional purposes (and for all the detail nuts out there), I did some research. What I found simply confirmed what I already knew from experience and observation—that this plan was good to go. I include the approximate (average) totals; there will be some variation, depending on what and how much you actually choose to eat.

I don't think a late snack is a good idea, but if you're having a real snack attack, eat a small bowl of cereal or a piece of toast with a little peanut butter. While it's not a great idea to eat before bed, you're better off having a small bowl of good cereal than a pint of Ben and Jerry's. What's a good cereal? Here's a good rule of thumb: A cartoon on the box = no good (read the label).

I personally don't usually eat between meals during the day. I find that I have more energy that way. But I realize that many people feel like they'll just collapse if they don't have some snacks in between meals or before they go to bed. That's why I added them to the menu. Just don't eat junk for a snack—it just defeats the purpose, don't you think?

Remember: Before you start this, please get your thinking right. Losing weight is not easy, and anyone who tells you that you aren't going to be hungry when trying to lose weight is blowing smoke up your butt. The eat-all-you-want-and-still-lose-weight line is nonsense, and it's amazing to me that anyone would believe it. The point here is to bear down on it till you reach your goal. Then you can loosen up on the plan a little and still keep your weight stable. It's not easy, but nothing worth having ever is.

If you honestly stay close to this plan and do the right PT, you should have no problem with your weight. Notice that I didn't give you many exact portion sizes or measurements. You don't need to sweat it so closely. It doesn't matter if you eat exactly a cup or a cup and a quarter cup of cereal. Nobody ever got fat by eating an extra quarter cup of Raisin Bran at breakfast, nor did they blow up because they ate eight ounces of grilled salmon instead of six. Use your half a brain here. It's the huge bag of chips or order of french fries with your lunch sandwich (or that big bowl of ice cream that you have before you go to bed) that gets you in trouble. It's common sense. If you're very active and working hard on the job, you can eat more, meaning more of the good stuff, like another good sandwich for lunch.

Now don't get mental. Nobody's going to take away your Girl Scout cookies or any other of your favorite foods—this is simply a plan. Many of you may not even need to follow this plan exactly to lose weight since everybody is different. You can switch lunch and dinner around if you need to. Just keep in mind that if you're trying to lose weight, you'll see better results the closer you stay to this plan. On this plan you may notice a quick weight loss of five pounds or so in the first week, but after that you should try to lose no more than two pounds a week. Any weight that comes off too quickly will go right back on just as quickly. DO NOT TAKE ANY FAT BURNERS OR ANY OTHER WEIGHT-LOSS SUPPLEMENTS, UNLESS THEY ARE PRESCRIBED BY A DOCTOR!

From my experience, if you're honest and are doing good PT, it's just about impossible to not lose weight on this plan. If you try to restrict your calories more than this, you won't be able to perform well on the job or otherwise. Plus, if you try to eat much less than this, you'll soon give up and pig out (just like you've probably done many times before). Think long-term and high-performance eating.

Tips for Military Personnel and First Responders

If you're a military person or a first responder, or maybe a working person who's putting in some extra overtime, you may have to miss regular meals because you're working an extended operation. In these cases, you need something you can grab and eat on the go. I've been in combat operations where getting something to eat was a hit-or-miss prospect. Yes, you can go a long way without food and sleep if you have to, but to work hard around the clock, think effectively, and prevent injury, you need to eat something at least every three to four hours. I'm not talking about your everyday routine here. During these high output times, it's all about performance, not trying to lose weight. You need to supplement your normal meal schedule with something that's easy and will keep you going. Another consideration is the fact that this type of work, to say the least, can be very stressful. Putting the wrong thing in an empty, stressed-out stomach can make you feel sick. I've been in these situations many times, and because of that I've tried just about every pre-packaged snack food out there. Protein and energy bars, jerky, dried fruit and nut mixes, different types of sports drinks, you name it.

In my opinion, the single best pre-made snack food to eat during these types of situations is a regular PowerBar. I like the peanut butter one, but the flavor is up to you as they all have about the same breakdown. It's unbreakable, packed with fast energy, easy to digest, and keeps well. Another thing I've always liked is that it doesn't melt all over the place in hot conditions like most of the other "coated" bars do. Plus, you can also find it just about everywhere. It goes down well with water and tastes great with coffee, which, in 99 out of 100 times, is the only thing you'll get to drink during these times (and to be honest, hot coffee will be a treat). I've never had a problem digesting it, even while eating it in the middle of running/biking during a triathlon. I've worked for days on end, with little time for regular meals, but PowerBars filled in the blanks and kept me going.

I realize that you may not like the taste of a PowerBar, but there are a lot of good protein and energy bars out there. Try different ones to find the ones that work for you. While I always try to eat regular, non-processed food, when you're super busy those bars are good to go. Lastly on sports bars, they're pretty dry in any case, so make sure you drink plenty of water with them.

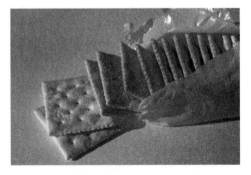

Two other good choices, but not always as practical as grabbing an energy bar, are regular old saltine crackers and the old school peanut butter and jelly sandwich. During my time on Navy ships, we often went through some very heavy seas, especially in the North Atlantic. People would be seasick, puking all over the place. The chow hall would put out big trays of saltine crackers for people to eat. The salt and the simple, non-greasy makeup of these crackers can help settle your stomach and keep you going. As you'd guess, they don't travel all that well but they do work.

Meal, Ready to Eat (MRE) crackers are basically the same thing and travel much better, but they don't taste all that great by themselves and are dry as hell. Same goes for pretzels. PBJ is good to go for people on the run; if you have the time to make it, it may be the best, quick pick-me-up. It's a good sandwich when traveling, too. Sounds too simple, huh? Not high-tech enough for you? Well, if you have some time to waste, do the nutritional breakdown of a PBJ sandwich on good whole-wheat bread—it's pretty close to what most energy bars contain (and can be better than many) at a fraction of the cost. In my book, a PBJ sandwich (natural peanut butter on whole-grain bread) also tastes better, especially if you can pop it in a microwave for 10–15 seconds.

I have also eaten a lot of trail mix and beef jerky during these times. Trail mix is good when hiking, especially during cooler weather, as it packs a lot of calories. Be sure to read the label, as many brands have a lot of sugar in them. Look for the mix that's mostly just plain dried fruit and nuts, not chocolate. I like beef jerky, but keep in mind that it's almost all protein and has nearly zero carbs. It's good to get the protein it provides, but when working long and hard, you'll need mostly carbs to keep you going. I would stay away from candy, however. Yes, it has plenty of carbs, but the high simple sugar content will spike your blood sugar and then you'll have an energy crash in about half an hour. The same goes for the liquid sugar: soda. Try different stuff to see what works best for you. I always keep PowerBars, trail mix, and beef jerky around. You never know what might come up.

During the evacuation and the following cleanup work from Hurricane Ivan in 2004, I ate a lot of those items and not much else. I was able to work in the very hot, extremely humid conditions, cutting trees and cleaning up the washed-up garbage with little else for the first few days. I'll admit I drank a few cold beers (we did have some ice) every night, and that didn't hurt, either.

There's no secret or miracle diet out there. No matter what the experts tell you, consistent effort in your PT program, combined with common-sense eating and a little patience, is the only answer to managing your weight. I always tell everyone to eat like an adult, and you know what I mean.

CHAPTER 9

EXCUSES, VAMPIRES, AND USELESS INFO

In this chapter, I want to go over a few things that are important to consider when you're planning a PT and eating routine. As I'm always about the thought process and getting your thinking right first, I think they need to be discussed. These are some odds and ends that aren't always talked about, but in my opinion they can make the difference between the success and failure of a program. More than anything else, they'll help you get your head screwed on right.

Excuses

During my 28 years of being a Marine, I was often assigned some hard tasks. They weren't always physical or required great courage. (In fact, I would've rather gone a few rounds with Mike Tyson than have to complete some of the administrative stuff I was given to do.) Later as moved into leadership positions, I was the one assigning tasks, and I learned that one key to help get a group of hard-headed people to do something they don't want to do is to take away their excuses. Essentially, it's 1,000 times better to deal with them right up front.

This little technique (when you have the time to do it) can save you time and headaches. That's why I'm going to take away your excuses of why you can't PT or eat right. I know you may have some excuses that I haven't heard of (and I've heard a bunch), but I'll address the most common.

"I don't have time! I'm too busy!"

This is probably the most common one, and in most cases it's just a load of bull. Time—that clock on the wall—is something we're all bound by. Got to get to work, pay the bills; got to get home, pick up the kids; got to get to class; etc. I live by it like everyone else. So why do some people always seem so busy, while others seem to get things done and still have some free time? I'll tell you why: Most people with this problem are simply not honest with themselves, are unorganized, and/or don't know how much time they waste every day.

Most people who say they don't have time to PT really do have the time. They just don't want to admit it, and in the end the time thing is just an easy, weak excuse. I can prove this with my trusty "Math for Marines" training. Last time I checked, there are 24 hours in day, 7 days in a week. That totals 168 hours in a week.

As I've already explained, you need only three to five hours a week of the right PT to get and stay in great shape. That's real shape, and that's about three percent of your total time (five hours). Now think about all the time you waste surfing the internet, watching TV, playing computer games, sitting at the bar, etc. See where I'm going here?

Be honest. If you're so busy that you can't dedicate three to five hours a week to improve your health, appearance, and overall outlook on life, then it's because you're in such dire straits money-wise that you have to work 24/7 to make ends meet. If that's really the case, you won't have time to read this book, let alone PT, so I say God bless you and good luck. I hope things turn around for you.

For the rest of you bullshit artists, you're not that busy. Most likely what you're doing is running around like a chicken with its head chopped off all day, then you come home and collapse in front of the idiot box or jump online for hours, wasting much more time than you think with mindless nonsense. I like TV like anyone else, even though I think most of it's garbage, and while I don't play video games, I do use the internet, but I just don't let it hypnotize me for hours on end. If you don't believe me, keep track of your TV, video game, and computer time for a week. It'll be more than you think.

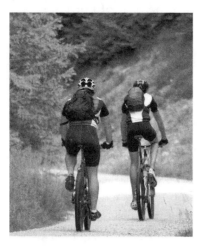

As far as no time to eat right? My friend, you're going to have to eat one way or another, and it takes just as much time to eat crap as it does to eat good food. You're not too busy—you're just wasting the time you need to get in shape, so get a grip.

"I'm too tired."

I touched briefly on this earlier, and I believe you're tired. Life will tire you out, especially if you have a very physical and/or stressful job. Being tired from a long, hard day of work is normal. That's why it's called work and why we don't do it for free. It doesn't matter if it's all physical or mostly mental. It'll all make you tired. However, being tired and too tired to do what you need and/or want to do are two different animals. Being overweight, out of shape, and eating a poor diet will make it much worse. Combine all that with a lifestyle of smoking, drinking too much, and the depression that normally follows with poor health and you're a time bomb waiting to go off. Actually, you're more like a weak bridge waiting to collapse. Forget just being tired; it's going to make you old, sick, and eventually drive you to an early grave. That's not just my opinion, it's a fact. I've seen it happen to friends and family all my life. You can do better.

You just need to get your head right and follow my (simple) guidance as far as PT goes, eat right, and you'll be surprised by what you can do. As you get into better condition and your weight gets to where it should be, your energy level will dramatically increase. You'll do more and feel less tired. Sorry, but the "I'm too tired to PT" excuse doesn't cut it with me, and you shouldn't let it with you, either.

"I don't have the money for a gym or expensive home equipment."

This one is all a matter of perspective. To get in great shape, you don't really need a gym or expensive home gear. You can get in shape without them. And no, I don't consider a set of kettlebells or a quality weighted vest expensive. They do cost a little bit, but they have a lot of real value. When I talk about expensive home gear, I'm talking about the rubber band and bow-and-arrow-type weightlifting machines you see on TV 24/7. They're the most expensive book and clothes racks I've ever seen because that's what most of them end up being. Try to find a set of used kettlebells for sale, but this may be hard to do because people tend to keep quality stuff that they use; useless junk, on the other hand, is always for sale. Think about it.

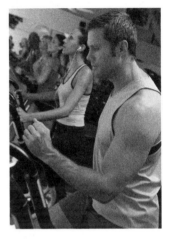

I've PT'ed in at least a hundred different gyms in my life, from huge modern facilities (some even had a full bar) to gyms that were nothing more than a prison exercise yard. I've also had my own home gym set-ups at different times. Based on that experience, I strongly feel that the cost of a membership to a good gym is well worth the price. A year's membership to a full-service fitness center is about the same cost as one of those foolish home fitness machines I was talking about. The gym membership is a much better investment, in my opinion. It's not the actual money you spend, as it's much less than some of the other garbage you'll waste money on. It's the value of what it can give you. What price would you put on your health and fitness?

Lately with the tough economy, I've seen some pretty good deals advertised for gym memberships. Another good angle is to look into supporting your local YMCA, Boys & Girls Club or community center. Many have good set-ups and are comparatively inexpensive. Plus, you'd be supporting your local business in the process, which is always a good thing.

"I have health problems that prevent me from exercising."

Before you start any exercise plan or diet, check in with your doctor. The guidance in this book is for people who are in generally good health and need/want to obtain a high level of fitness. However, as always, be honest with yourself. I've seen some people with poor health and disabilities do pretty impressive things over the years. Also, if you're a military member or a first responder and aren't in decent enough health to PT? No offense, but maybe you shouldn't be on that job in the first place.

"PT is boring. I can't get anyone to work out with me."

Hello, you're not five years old and need to be entertained 24/7. Exercise by its nature has to be repetitious to be effective. Again, you aren't exercising for social reasons. I've worked out with many people over the years and have had both great and bad experiences. Having a friend to PT with can be fun and an advantage. They can motivate you when you don't feel like going and are tired, etc. However, overall, if I had to choose between the two, I'd rather PT by myself because this is *my* time. It's about getting MY butt in shape. You need to motivate yourself from the inside on this. If you rely on someone else too much for motivation, in the end you'll fail to reach your goals.

In the end, it's too much hassle to worry about another person when working out. They're often late, or don't show up at all. They want to change your routine. That may sound selfish and harsh, and it may be—but so what? Remember what I said about "results"? Results are the goal here, not being social. You'll have plenty of time to hang with your friends. If you're having trouble being alone with yourself for about an hour a day, get yourself an iPod, load it up with your favorite tunes, and you'll be fine.

I could go on and on with excuses why you can't do this. The bottom line here is that if you really want to get in shape and get your weight right, you'll find the time. The time and energy is there if you just open your eyes and look, I promise. Change your thinking. Instead of looking for reasons not to go, start looking at your schedule and see where you can fit in a PT. Like everything else, it all starts or stops with the thought process.

Vampires

This is not about the monsters you see in the movies. This is about vampires you see every day. You know them—they're at your work, the gym, or anywhere that you may hang out. These vampires don't drink your blood. What they do is much worse: They suck the life force from you. These people, including family and friends, are probably good people for the most part, but a five-minute conversation with them is like swimming the English Channel. You can actually be physically tired from just talking to them.

These vampires often travel in groups with two other anti-superheroes, "Negative Man" (or "Negative Woman") and trusty sidekick "Duty Expert." Negative Man has only one super power, which is to put the worst possible spin on any situation—nothing is good, everything and everybody is bad; only the worst things are sure to happen and everybody is out to get you. "You can't win, so why bother" is his motto. This is especially true about anything that you may attempt in the area of getting yourself in shape, losing weight, or eating right. Negative Man will always warn you about the dangers of running too much and eating too little. He might also take a completely opposite view, depending on which is the most negative at the time. He thrives on failure, doom, gloom, and horrible endings. But he has one weakness. His kryptonite is a happy smile, a motivated attitude, and, above all else, a positive outlook. Deliver these anywhere near Negative Man and he'll quickly flee the scene or dissolve on the spot. In fact, he'll try to avoid you in the future, once he realizes you display any optimistic traits.

His buddy "Duty Expert" is always ready to give you the benefit of his vast knowledge. He knows all and has done all. Only by following his exact guidance could you succeed in achieving your goals. Or should I say his goals, as your goals can only be what he determines are the right goals. If he didn't think of them, they aren't worth pursuing. However, he also has an Achilles heel. Duty Expert lives for the argument, the slightest challenge to his expertise. Thus his downfall is agreement and a sincere thanks for his advice (but just don't really take it). Without a point to prove, he'll quickly move to another person who needs his mentorship. For when you publicly acknowledge his superior experience and know-how, he cannot afford to waste any more time on you, not while there are so many others deserving and needing of his time and talent. Negative Man and Duty Expert normally do their best work from a bar stool, behind a cloud of cigarette smoke, and in between bites of french fries.

Now what's all this BS? It's just a funny way to just warn you that many people in your life will try to undermine your efforts to get in shape and lose weight. They'll tell you that working out is a waste of time, the program you're doing won't work, you'll get hurt, you're too old, etc. I've personally heard it many, many times in my life. Just put in some effort, have some faith, and great results will follow. There's always somebody out there to tell you you can't do something. What they really mean is *they* can't do it. So just blow them off and keep going. To be honest, these people have always motivated me to train harder, so I guess I drain them of their energy in the end.

Useless Info

I close out this book with some useless info. Not that it isn't good—it's great advice. It's useless because any sane adult should already know this stuff, and the other reason is the fact that you'll either do it or you won't. It doesn't matter what I say one way or the other. Like I used to tell officers I worked for over the years, "Sir, you may choose to ignore my advice. That's your choice. However, you're going to hear it regardless."

Doing drugs, drinking too much, and smoking cigarettes (like your lungs are on fire) WILL keep you from getting in shape, and eventually ruin your health. We all know people who smoke and drink but still look ok, and I've seen some who can PT pretty well. That won't last. As General Grant used to say about the Confederacy hanging tough in the Civil War with limited soldiers and supplies, "They can't beat the math"—meaning at some point those bad habits WILL catch up with you. It's not a matter of "if," either. Do yourself a favor: Quit smoking and keep your drinking under control. If you're doing drugs, you need to get some help ASAP. To be honest, I seriously doubt if anyone who had enough interest in getting in shape to buy this book would be an alcoholic or drug user. However, you never know so I'm throwing it out there.

Lastly, do yourself a BIG favor: Relax when you can. Like myself, I'll bet many of the people reading this book are Type A personalities—driven, ambitious, and many times impatient and short-tempered workaholics. There's a price to all that internal fire: stress. Stress can make you stronger, just like increased exercise, but it has been shown to be bad for your health, especially in the long term. PT can really help to bleed off some steam from the pressure cooker. I can be a real jerk on days I don't get to PT (ask my family). I think it's more of an attitude shift than anything else. Some things you just have to let go as they're just not worth getting upset about. Easier said than done, I realize, but I guarantee PT will help.

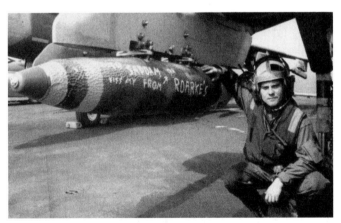

The author at work during Desert Storm.

One thing I've learned to do (or try, at least) is to separate myself from things that get me spooled up. For example, most of my life I was a news junkie; I used to love the 24-hour cable news shows. During Desert Storm, I was deployed on a Navy ship and saw very little news for eight months. What happened? Nothing. I missed the constant news updates at first, but I was pretty busy. In the end, it showed me that 99 percent of the stuff that seemed so important really wasn't. The world didn't end because I missed the latest news. I still like to keep up with what's going on, but at a much reduced time investment. Try it and you'll be amazed by how little you miss it. The same goes for e-mail 24/7.

Lastly, when I was younger I got in fist fights all the time. I got my ass kicked a few times, but I kicked plenty, too. However, the outcome didn't really matter that much to me; I just wanted to prove how tough I was and get some respect (whatever that means). Most of the fights were over something stupid (like they always are).

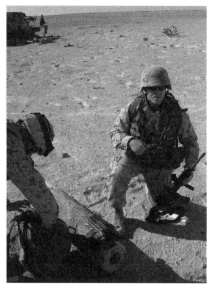
Iraq, 2005.

In the mid-1980s, I was on a deployment to Fallon, Nevada. One night at the enlisted club, a bigger, higher-ranked Marine was messing with one of my junior Marines, so like a idiot I busted him in his mouth. Bad move all around—he went down and cracked his head on the sidewalk. He ended up in the hospital and I ended up in the brig. I almost threw my career down the drain with that one punch. My leadership took up for me, and I managed to not to get into serious trouble. Since he could've died from the head injury, I could've gone to prison. I don't know where I'd be today if that had happened. What I learned from that incident? Everybody loses in a fight over nonsense.

The main point I'm making is to find some things to do in your life that don't have to be done at a million miles an hour, that don't have a bar to jump over. What are things that you like to do without any goals you have to reach for? Having the ability to really relax can go a long way to keeping you healthy and getting some fun out of life. For all the work you do for other people, you deserve it. Be safe and good luck.

Semper Fi
Master Gunz

APPENDICES

SAT TIME BREAKDOWN

In Chapter 4, I gave you the standard breakdown for a one-hour SAT workout. To recap:

1) Warm-up: 5 minutes

2) Pre-Fatigue: 30 minutes

3) Mission: 20 minutes

4) Cool-down: 5 minutes

However, sometimes you won't have a full hour (you may be tired, lack time, or are working your way up to the full hour) but still want to get in a workout. So I've designed two shorter sessions, one that's 30 minutes (Level I) and another that's 45 (Level II). To be honest, you could get, and stay, in some pretty decent shape with Level II workouts only, but the extra 15 minutes that take you up to a full hour-long session will add a lot to your conditioning.

As you do these SAT workouts, you'll quickly develop a sense of what you can get done in the time you have. I put together these routines so that you can get a balanced PT session in the time allotted. Obviously, the better condition you're in, the more you'll be able to accomplish, so add or subtract as needed. To do a Support session in any of these times, keep the warm-up and cool-down the same and do whatever activity you would normally do for a Support workout, just in a shorter time frame.

Level I > Total time: 30 minutes

Warm-up	5 minutes (the same warm-up is always used; see page 108)
Pre-Fatigue	10 minutes
Mission	10 minutes
Cool-down	5 minutes (the same cool-down is always used; see page 112)

Don't let the short amount of time fool you—you can get a serious workout in 30 minutes. This is what I recommend if you're first starting out with EPRS, or if you're tired or short on time. Always do the same warm-up and cool-down. Don't shorten them; you'll risk injury if you do. For the Pre-Fatigue, just do any of your normal pre-fatigue activities but limit it to ten minutes. As for the Mission, I recommend you do 10 minutes of non-weight movements (calisthenics) since 10 minutes is really not enough time to get the weights going. I often use this quick workout when I'm traveling and don't have time to locate or go to a full-service gym.

Here are a few examples. Any of these will be a serious workout for 10 minutes, and overall this is about as good a workout as you can get for 30 minutes.

Do 1 cycle of 3 fast rotations; repetition goals are in parentheses.

1. Any pull-up (10–15), free squats (15–25), any push-up (25–50), any abs (50+)
2. Any pull-up (10–15), 8 counts (5–10), any push-up (25–50), any abs (50+)
3. Any pull-up (10–15), step-ups (5–10), any push-up (25–50), any abs (50+)

Level II > Total time: 45 minutes

Warm-up	5 minutes
Pre-Fatigue	20 minutes
Mission	15 minutes
Cool-down	5 minutes

At this point, I think you can figure out how to do a 20-minute Pre-Fatigue. For Level II (15-minute) Mission workouts, do the same cycles as the full 1-hour workout, but just do two rotations of each of the first 3 cycles and 1 set of the last cycle.

EXERCISE GLOSSARY

PULL-UPS

Regular Pull-Ups

This is the classic, basic pull-up. The width of your grip can vary from shoulder width to very wide. I suggest you vary this width during your workouts to keep your body guessing.

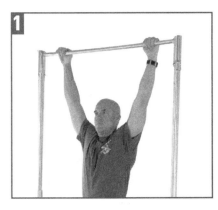 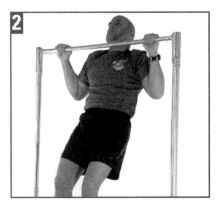

1 Place your hands about shoulder-width apart on a pull-up bar with your palms facing away from you. All your fingers should be on the same side of the bar. If needed, cross your feet to help prevent excessive body motion.

2 From a "dead hang," pull up till your chin is over the bar, and then lower all the way back down for one rep.

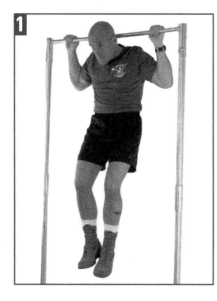

Behind-the-Neck Pull-Ups

For behind-the-neck pull-ups, widen your grip slightly more than regular pull-ups. You'll have to experiment till you find the right width that is comfortable for you. These are the hardest of all pull-ups, and will really add to your back development.

1 Grasp the bar in the same manner as in regular pull-ups. If needed, cross your feet to help prevent excessive body motion. Pull yourself up, placing the bar behind your neck by touching the bar at the base of your neck. Lower all the way down for one rep.

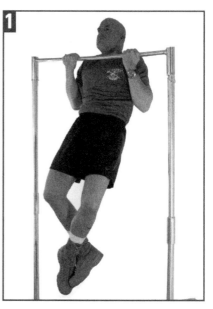

Chin-Ups

This pull-up provides the most direct workout for your biceps, more than any of the other pull-ups.

1 Grasp the bar with your palms facing you, about shoulder-width apart. Cross your feet to help prevent excessive body motion. Pull yourself up till your chin is over the bar, and then lower all the way down for one rep.

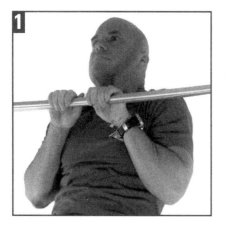

Close-Grip Pull-Ups

This pull-up will condition the pulling muscles in the center of your back.

1 Grasp the bar with your hands together (thumbs touching), palms facing away from you. Cross your feet to help prevent excessive body motion. Pull your chin over the bar and lower down for one rep.

Commando Pull-Ups

Commando pull-ups start with your body aligned length-wise with the bar.

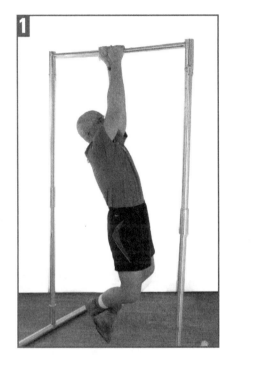 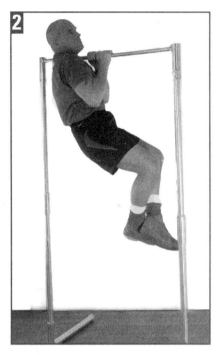

1 Grasp the bar with your hands, touching one in front of the other. Cross your feet to help prevent excessive body motion.

2 Pull yourself up, moving your head around to one side of the bar until your shoulder touches the bar. Lower for one rep. For each rep, alternate your head movement from one side to the other. Also for each set, alternate the hand that is in front of your grip. These need to be done slowly and with control to prevent excessive swinging.

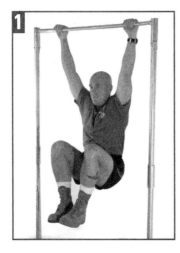

V-Ups

V-ups are a great way to combine some abdominal work with pull-ups. These are also very good for conditioning your grip.

1 Grasp the bar as in regular pull-ups and execute a regular pull-up (see page 81). After you lower, raise your knees to your chest and then lower them again. Count the completion of both movements as one rep.

You can vary this by doing up to 5 (or more) knee raises in between each pull-up. You can also do these with behind-the-neck pull-ups (good luck with that, stud). The pause and lifting action needed to do the knee raises in between the pull-ups will really work your grip strength/endurance. I do these all the time, as they're one of my favorite movements.

Pull-Downs

I've listed these in the pull-up section as they work the same muscles. While I do pull-ups and push-ups almost every work-out, I'd say that at least once a week I substitute the lat pull-down machine at the gym for pull-ups. These can be done with many different grip methods, including a rope end. These machines are simple to use and easy to understand. However, if you've never used these before, I suggest that you get someone working at the gym (trainer/manager) to show you how to properly set up and use the machine. I've seen some pretty good improvement in pull-up ability made by Marines using these machines.

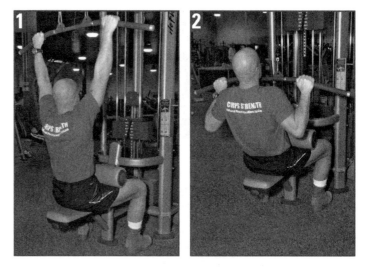

1 Before you start, adjust the hold-down pad into the correct position over your legs so that it'll firmly hold your body in place, but without being too tight. Choose a weight that will allow you to get at least 15 reps, better 20. When working with this machine, it's better to do more reps than you'd normally get with standard pull-ups. This allows you to work on developing the upper range of your max pull-ups.

2 Ensure you perform along the full range of movement and concentrate on executing smooth, controlled repetitions. Don't jerk or let the weights freefall back.

Assisted Pull-Ups

If you can't do many, or any, pull-ups on your own (especially the behind-the-neck version), you can still make progress by using a couple of different methods. All these do is reduce the actual amount of weight that you're pulling. If you can't get 5 strict reps on your own, you should add a few assisted reps to the end of each set. As a last resort, if you have no training partner or chair available, you can "kip" (slightly swing) yourself over the bar and then very strictly and slowly lower yourself down. The slow descent will help develop the strength in your arms and back needed to do pull-ups. Pull-ups are a tough exercise and will take time and effort to improve. To be honest, if you're overweight, one of the best (quickest) ways to increase your pull-ups is to lose excess body fat. It can make a huge difference. I've seen this many times with Marines. So be patient.

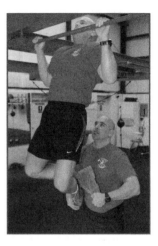

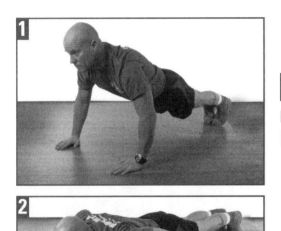

PUSH-UPS

Regular Push-Ups

1 Place your hands on the floor a little wider than shoulder-width apart, with your fingers facing forward (if they turn outward a little, that's ok). Keep your feet together; your weight should only be supported by your toes and your hands. Keep your head up, looking forward, and your back straight.

2 Lower down until your arms are bent parallel to the floor, then press back up to complete one rep.

Wide Push-Ups

The wide push-up is performed just like the regular push-up, except with hands placed farther apart. This can vary from anything beyond the normal width to very wide. Try different widths during your workouts. I find that the wider I go with my stance, the more I need to turn my hands outward to make it comfortable for my shoulders. Try it and figure out what works best for you.

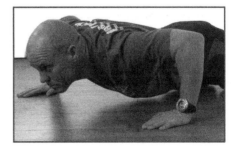

Incline Push-Ups

Incline push-ups are really just like any of the other types of push-ups, but you do them with your feet elevated off the ground. The degree of incline can be varied (and should be) from just slightly elevated on a step to very steeply on a high bench. This puts more work on your shoulders, which makes the push-up harder since your body weight is more focused on your arms rather than divided between your feet and arms. These are one of my favorites, and especially tough while wearing a weighted vest.

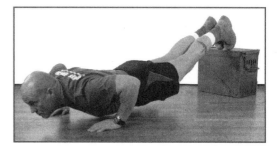

Diamond Push-Ups

Diamond push-ups are named such because you place your hands together in a diamond shape. This tough movement focuses more on your triceps than other push-ups. It's important to note that, because you're using

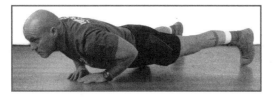

a very narrow hand stance, it's best to spread your legs to provide better balance. A key factor is where you place your body weight, meaning where your weight is centered over your hands. You really have to find your own "sweet spot" on this. You'll know it's not right because it'll hurt your shoulders.

Dips

Dips are a more advanced version of the push-up. The best place to do these is on a dip station, which is two bars/pipes that are spread a short distance apart, about four feet or so off the ground.

1 Place one hand on each bar, with your thumbs on the same side as your other fingers. Keep your arms straight.

2 Keeping your head up and looking straight ahead, lower your body till your elbows are just below parallel. Push back up to complete one rep. You really don't need to go below parallel on this movement; in fact, it would be better to go a little short rather than below parallel. In my opinion, going below parallel puts too much stress on your shoulder joints and has little added benefit.

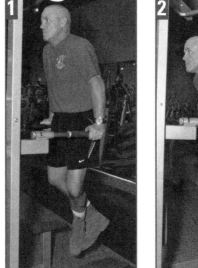
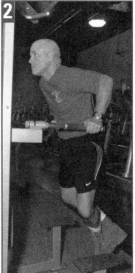

Mountain Climber Push-Ups

This is a combination of mountain climbers and push-ups, combining a strength exercise (push-ups) with a more aerobic movement (mountain climbers). I like exercise movements that condition both your strength and your endurance at the same time because, in real-life challenges, those are likely to be the requirements.

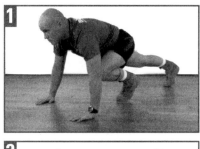

1 Start in the push-up position, but bring your left knee up to your chest. Now bring your right knee to your chest and extend your left leg back. Perform 1–5 mountain climbers by quickly alternating your legs back and forth; two leg movements equal one rep. Keep your head up and eyeballs off the doggone deck.

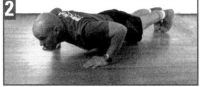

2 Once you've done 1–5 mountain climbers, lower into a regular push-up (see page 85). From the up position, continue doing mountain climbers.

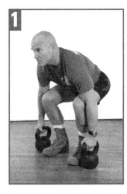

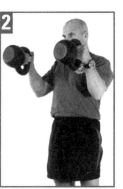

WHEEL-HOUSE

Deadlift Curl

1 Squat and grasp two kettlebells/or dumbbells. Make sure that your butt is below your knees, your back is straight, and your head is up and looking forward.

2 Stand up. From here, curl the weights up to your chest and then back down. This is one rep. Start the next rep by squatting to where your weights slightly touch the ground and, without stopping, come right back up.

Squat Press

1 Grasp one kettlebell/dumbbell/ammo can and place it at your chest, right under your chin. Squat down until your butt is at least below parallel.

2 Come back up. When you're fully straight, press the weight overhead and then bring it back down for a rep. The key to this is to try and not pause at any one place in the exercise; keep your movements fluid. This will get you breathing hard very quickly.

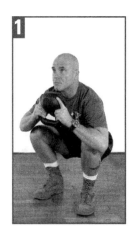

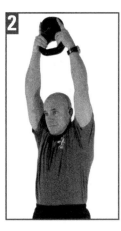

APPENDIX B: EXERCISE GLOSSARY **87**

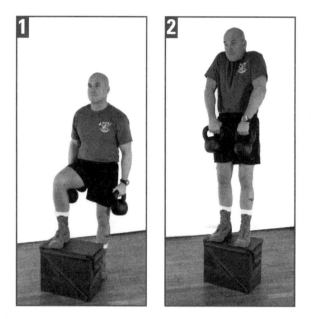

Step-Up Shrug

I developed this exercise as it simulates a real-life movement, specifically for military personnel or fire-fighters. Many times when you carry something up stairs or a hill, once you get there you have to throw it up on a truck, table, ledge, etc. This exercise conditions you for the situation.

1 Grasp your choice of weight in your hands and step up on something (anything stable of about a foot or so in height).

2 Once you have both feet on the step, "shrug" the weight as high as you can. This means raising the weight using your neck and shoulder muscles, not by bending your arms. This is a short movement of about 6–8 inches but strengthens the most important part of any upward lift—the initial upward motion.

Lateral Swing

The lateral swing can be done with almost any weight you can firmly grasp with one hand, but it's best done with kettlebells because you can perform a hand exchange during the movement.

1 Holding the weight in one hand, squat down with the weight between your legs.

2 Stand up as you swing the weight forward and up. The upward movement should end when the weight is an arm's length above and in front of your head, and you've stood all the way up. *If you're using kettlebells*, switch hands at the point just before the weight starts back down. Come back down to the squat position for one rep. *If you're using a dumbbell or an ammo can*, I recommend using both hands and not switching hands.

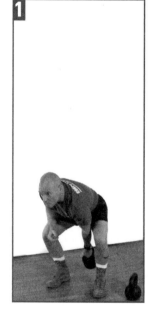
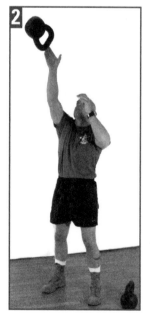

Rowing (One-Arm)

Probably no movement is better for conditioning real-life working muscles than rowing, which develops your back and arm strength together. It can be done several different ways.

When doing the one-armed version, stand with one arm braced either on your knee, a bench, or on the handle of another weight. Bend over and draw your weight from the ground up to your chest, and then lower back down for one rep. Switch arms and repeat.

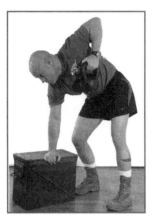

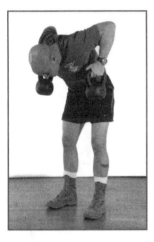

Rowing (Two-Arm)

When using both arms at the same time, the important point is to brace your stance in a way that will provide a powerful position in which to draw the weights upward without straining your back. Again, draw your weights up to your chest then lower back down for one rep.

Rowing (Cable)

In a gym I like to use the cable rowing machine, the kind where you brace your feet and pull a weight stack up with a cable. While you can use many different attachment grips, I like to use the close grip, as it's more realistic. It's important here to keep your back straight, head up, and control the weight throughout the full range of the movement. I think this is one of the best gym machines to use to build working fitness.

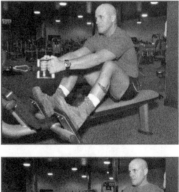

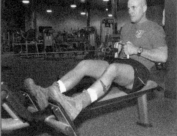

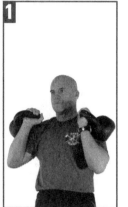 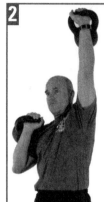

Overhead Press

This a classic exercise. It can also be done with two arms at a time.

1 Grasp your weights and clean them up to your shoulders. Make sure that you have a solid stance as you do this.

2 From here, press the weight overhead and lower back down for one rep. This is a good movement to use one big kettlebell if you have one. If you're using two smaller weights, either press them up together or alternate left and right arms.

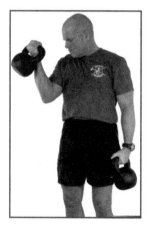

Curls

Curls develop your grip and the pulling power of your arms. They can be done several different ways.

From a standing position, hold the weights along your sides with your palms facing inward. As you curl the weights to your chest, twist your palms so that they're facing you. You can curl both arms at the same time or alternate arms.

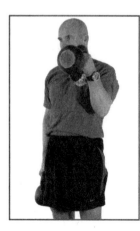

Hammer Curls

To do a hammer curl, grasp the weight with the handle facing upward. This is especially tough when using kettlebells.

Cable Curls

In the gym, you can use the cable curling machine, which is just a handle attached to a cable that pulls up a weight stack. This is a good curling exercise as the machine provides equal tension throughout the movement.

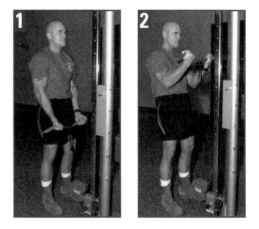

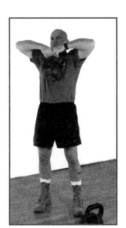
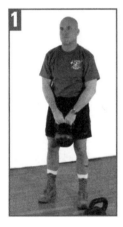

Upright Row

Upright rowing is another very important conditioning exercise. It conditions you for the everyday movement of raising something up from your waist to shoulder height. Do this with either one arm or two, a weight or a cable.

1 Grasp the weight at your waist while standing. Maintain a solid stance. Raise the weight to about chin height, and lower back down for one rep. Concentrate on smooth movement both up and down.

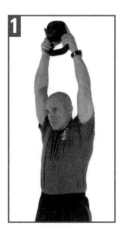

Front Raise

This is another good exercise for shoulder strength.

1 Grasp a dumbbell or kettlebell at your waist. Keeping your arms almost straight (without locking your elbows), raise the weight up to a position over your head. Lower slowly for one rep.

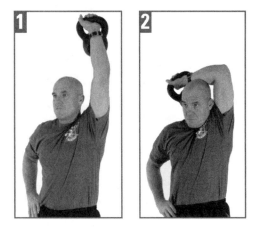

Triceps Press (Dumbbell)

This can be done while seated, but it provides better overall body conditioning if you perform it while standing. This can also be performed with both arms at the same time (with both hands on the same dumbbell/kettlebell). Just make sure that both elbows are kept straight overhead.

1 Take a dumbbell or kettlebell above your head, keeping your elbows straight.

2 Lower the weight toward the back of your head while keeping your elbow up. Go all the way down and back up overhead for one rep.

Triceps Press (Cable)

1 When using the triceps cable machine, hold your elbows close to your body.

2 Push the handle down till your arms are fully extended. Raise back up for one rep. The key to this movement is to position your body so that you put the full force of your tricep power downward, and to control the motion throughout the entire range of the movement.

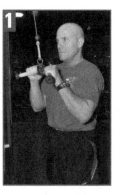
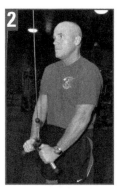

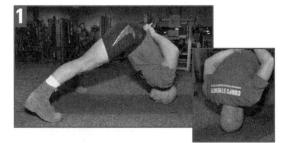

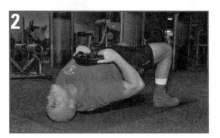

NECK EXERCISES

Neck Bridges

This is a great exercise (and my all-time-favorite neck movement) but one that you have to build up to.

1 Lie on your stomach and raise up on your forehead and toes. If you haven't done this before, keep your knees on the ground first to take some weight off your neck and get a feel for the movement. You can also place your hands on the ground near your head to provide some support. Slowly roll on your forehead in all possible directions.

2 After about a minute of so, flip over on your back and reverse the movement. The best place to do this is on an exercise or wrestling mat. GO SLOW!

Neck Curls

This is a good neck movement to do when you're in a gym. You can also do this outside with a kettlebell/dumbbell on any bench or bleacher you can lie down on.

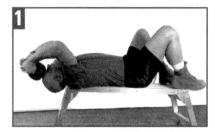

1 Get a plate of 10–25 pounds (or more; I use a 35-pound plate). Fold a towel and place it on the plate where it'll make contact with your forehead. Lie on a bench with your head over the side.

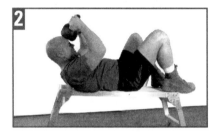

2 Rest the weight on your forehead and, using your hands to balance the weight, slowly lower the weight up and down. Make sure that you're only moving your neck, not your body, to "curl" the weight.

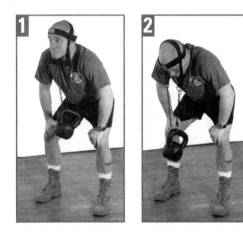

Neck Harness

1 Connect a kettlebell, dumbbell, or ammo can to a standard neck harness. Place the harness on your head and position yourself so that you can brace your hands against your knees.

2 Lower and raise the weight with your neck. Do the movement slowly to keep the weight from swinging excessively.

Neck Machine

Many gyms have a neck machine of some type, and there are many variations. (In my opinion, the Nautilus brand is the best.) If you haven't used one before, get someone at your gym to show you how. The most important aspect of using a neck machine is adjusting the seat to exactly the right height for your use. You'll need to figure this out through trial and error.

8 Counts

This Parris Island favorite can be a tough exercise. It's called 8 Counts because it has 8 separate movements to get one rep (though the pictures don't show all 8). It'll get you breathing hard in a hurry.

1 From a standing position, drop into a full squat with your hands on the ground.

2 Extend your legs out behind you in a high push-up position.

3 Lower down into the push-up.

4 Push yourself back up. Spread your legs apart and return them together.

5 Bring your legs back into the squat position as in step 1.

6 Stand back up to finish one rep.

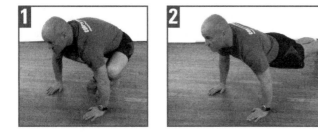

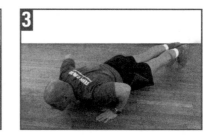

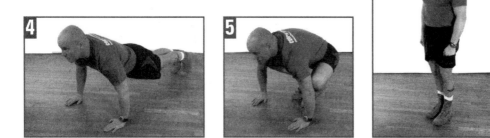

Free Squats

These are "free" in that you don't have to carry any weights (although it doesn't mean you can't use your weight vest).

1 From a standing position, squat down to at least where your butt is below parallel and extend your arms out for balance. You can go into a full squat if you'd like; just don't bounce at the bottom.

2 Stand back up and bring your arms back to your sides. To help with your balance, keep your back straight and your head up and look forward. The best way is to fix your gaze on a stationary object as you go up and down.

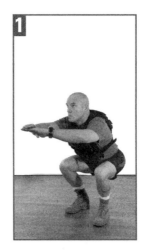
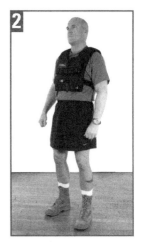

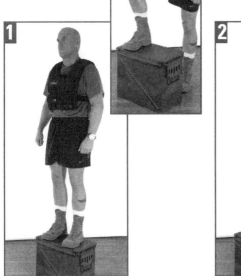
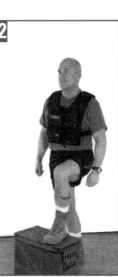

Step-Ups

Step-ups can be performed on anything stable that's 8–12 inches in height (you can go higher if you'd like).

1 Simply step up with one foot and then the other.

2 Step down with the same foot that you started with. The next rep starts with the other foot. Stepping up and down with both feet completes one rep.

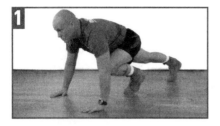

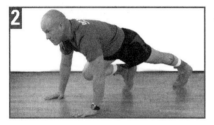

Mountain Climbers

This is one of my drill instructor's favorite rewards for privates (basically everyone) who didn't move fast enough for him.

1 Start in the push-up up position, but bring your left knee up to your chest.

2 Now bring your right knee to your chest and extend your left leg back. Perform the exercise by quickly alternating your legs back and forth. Keep your head up and your eyeballs off the doggone deck. Four leg movements equal one rep. For these, I always use the classic Marine Corps "four-count!" method to count the movements: 1, 2, 3, one! 1, 2, 3, two! Marines always do more with less.

GRIP

Wrist Curls

1 Stand with the weights along your sides and slowly open your hands, allowing the weights to lower toward your fingertips. Go as far as you can without dropping the weights.

2 Close your grip and the weights will rise upward into your palms. This completes one rep. This is the way your grip really works to hold items as you carry them.

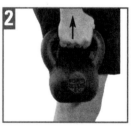

Wrist Roller

You can either make one of these or find one in a gym. It's basically a piece of rope that attaches to the center of something like a broomstick or pipe. The other end is attached to a weight of some type. Grabbing the device with your hands shoulder-width apart and keeping your elbows tight against your body, roll the weight up the rope till it's all the way to the handle. Slowly let it back down for a rep. You can do this quickly for a real forearm burn.

Grip Machine

Many gyms have some type of grip machine. Get someone in your local gym to show you how to use it properly.

Gripper

There are many different types of portable grippers. I've tried many of them and think that the "rock climber's doughnut" by Grip Pro Trainer is the best out there. One reason is that you can carry it everywhere. It also allows you to strengthen not only your overall grip but your individual fingers in just about any possible direction.

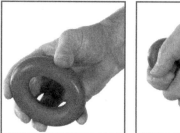 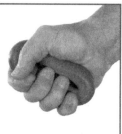

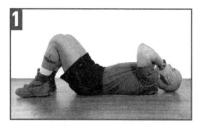

ABDOMINALS

Regular Crunch

1 Lie on your back with your feet flat on the ground and curled up almost to your butt. Place your fingers lightly against your ears.

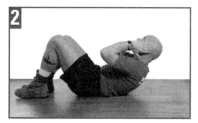

2 Curl your body upward to tighten your abdominal muscles. This is actually a very short movement of only a few inches. To get it right, you have to go by the way the tension feels in your stomach muscles. The key is to bring your head up just enough to completely tense your muscles; from that point you only have to raise a little more to complete the forward motion. Relax back down for one rep.

Flutter Kicks

When possible, I like to do this with my legs over the edge of a bench as it extends the range of my movement by letting me lower my legs below my body.

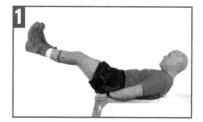

1 Lie on your back with your hands under your butt, keeping your knees slightly bent. Raise your feet about 45 degrees off the ground.

2 Alternately scissor your legs up and down. This can be done quickly. A full rotation of each leg is one rep.

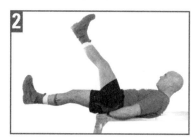

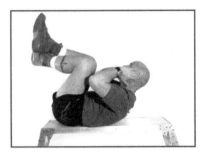

Elevated Crunch

Perform this like a regular crunch, but curl your legs up off the ground to hit your abdominals from a different angle.

Hello Dollies

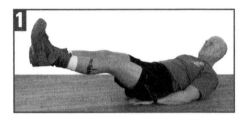

1 Lie on your back with your hands under your butt, keeping your knees slightly bent. Raise your feet about 45 degrees off the ground.

2 Keeping your legs elevated at all times, open and close your legs for one rep.

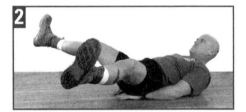

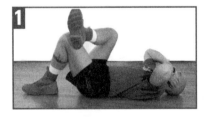

Side Crunches

1 Lie on your back with your feet flat on the ground. Cross your right leg over your left leg and place your fingers lightly against your ears.

2 Curl your body upward and move your left elbow toward your right knee. You should feel this more on one side of your abs. After a set amount of reps, switch legs and repeat on the other side.

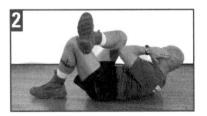

Leg Lifts

You can do this on an elevated bench rather than the ground. A bench will allow you to lower your legs past the level of your body, giving you a better stretch and range of movement.

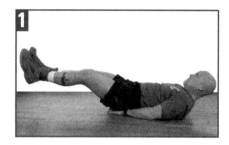

1 Lie on your back with your hands under your butt. Raise your head and shoulders off the ground.

2 Keeping your feet together, quickly raise your legs till they're at least level with your eyesight. Moving slowly and with control, lower them back down for a rep.

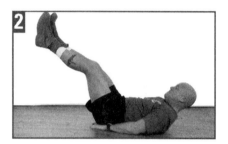

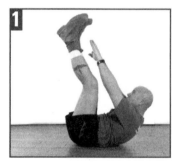

Reach Crunches

1 Lie on your back and raise your legs till they're almost straight up and down. Keep your feet together. Reach up with your arms and "crunch" forward and upward, reaching for your toes. The right "feel" will tell you if you're doing the movement correctly. Up and back down is one rep.

PRE-FATIGUE RUNNING WORKOUTS

As with all Pre-Fatigue sessions, your time limit is 30 minutes. However, with running you can also use 3 miles as a goal, stopping at whichever comes first. Here are some samples, performed on a standard quarter-mile track with a goal of varying the intensity within the 30 minutes. Of course, your Pre-Fatigue workouts don't need to be done on a track—if you're running down a road or a trail, you can sprint from any point you see (like telephone poles, trees, etc.), alternating with jogging or walking. You can also use a rowing machine, a spinning bike, etc. In any case, the most effective way to make your 30 minutes of Pre-Fatigue work is to constantly change and push yourself over different intervals within the time limit. Use your imagination and come up with your own. Of course, there'll be days when you're tired and you may just want to go out and jog 30 minutes, and that's fine, too.

A. Start slowly and increase speed for a total of 12 laps (3 miles) or 30 minutes, whichever comes first. Your goal is to complete 3 miles in less than 30 minutes, and then after that to reduce time. Three miles in 30 minutes is a very reasonable goal for anyone. Get close, or beat 20 minutes (wearing boots) for stud status.

B. Start slowly and run 1 mile at a moderate pace. At the start of the 2-mile mark, run 1 mile as fast as possible (less than 8 minutes is a good goal, 6 minutes for studs). Then jog the last mile, or when you get to 30 minutes. This is a good workout to increase 5k/10k speed.

C. Jog a ½ mile.

Run the next ½ mile at a hard pace, with a goal of less than 4 minutes. Stud status is less than 3 minutes.

Jog a ¼ mile.

Run a ½ mile at a hard pace.

Jog a ¼ mile.

Run a ½ mile at a hard pace.

Jog a ½ mile for a total of 3 miles or till you reach 30 minutes.

For another version, reverse the ½ and ¼ miles by sprinting the ¼ and jogging the ½. This is another good session for 5k/10k speed.

D. Jog 1 mile. Then for the next 2 miles sprint the straight parts and jog the curves. Do this for a total of 12 laps or until you reach 30 minutes. This a good routine to develop short sprinting speed, like that needed for touch football and softball. *For this workout, make sure you're thoroughly warmed up and ease into and out of full speed. It's easy to pull a hamstring with short, hard sprints. Trust me on this—I've been there.*

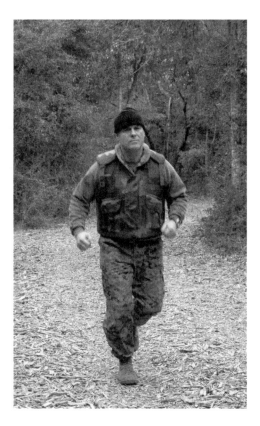

WEIGHTED VEST PT

Here are three basic weighted vest workouts for you to try out. They're all good, tough workouts, and there's no end to the variations you can come up with to make them harder. However, if you've never worked out with a weighted vest, you need to ease into it. It's a completely different thing but, I think, a valuable training tool for working people. I shouldn't have to say this but I will: Make sure you wear boots for any weighted vest workout. Running shoes will not cut it when carrying this extra weight. As with everything I recommend, adjust, improve, and tailor your workouts to your individual needs, goals, and conditioning.

A. Gym with a Stair Climber (or Stairs Nearby)

The Candidate Physical Ability Test (CPAT) requirement for the stair climber is 60 steps per minute for 3 minutes; this is done while wearing a 50-pound vest plus 25 pounds of additional weight to simulate a rescue pack or hose reel—75 pounds total. This is a serious load, trust me. If you're a firefighter who has to take the CPAT (or something similar) as an initial or annual testing requirement, then you'll need a vest that will hold 75 pounds. V-Max makes a vest that has a 25-pound weighted section that goes on and off, so you can go from 50 to 75 pounds easily. For everyone else, I think that 50 pounds is plenty to train with.

1. Warm up as usual without the vest.

2. Put on your vest and go to the stair climber. (NOTE: When using the stair climber, you have to practice/learn not to hold on to the rail or any other support as this is the requirement of the CPAT test.) Your goal is to work up to the normal Pre-Fatigue workout of 30 minutes. If you're using the full 75 pounds, I'd say that 10 minutes with that weight is enough because I think having the ability to triple the CPAT requirement is plenty in my book. If you feel up to it, you could do the whole 30 minutes with 75 pounds, but my gut feeling is that beyond 10 minutes, you're risking injury. Sixty steps a minute is really not that fast; it's a steady deliberate walk, but

"slow" is relative when carrying that much extra weight up stairs. Increase the speed of the climb if you like, but don't get crazy here. If you stumble (like my clumsy ass does once in a while) carrying 75 pounds of weight, you could very easily injure yourself. As always, train smart as well as hard. *Note:* You can use any regular stairs if you don't have access to a stair climber. Many public parks, especially in hilly regions, have stairs going from one part to another. Outdoor sports and entertainment stadiums have stairs, and you can find the same thing at most college and high-school stadiums. To be honest, I prefer this myself as it's outside and less boring than a stair-climbing machine. However, if you have to take the CPAT, you'll have to find a stair climber at some point to test your ability on the machine.

If you're not a firefighter preparing for CPAT testing and you're using 50 pounds or less in your vest, then it's ok to stay on the stair climber for your full 30 minutes. Just don't bust your ass if you can help it.

3. If you decide (and this is what I recommend if you're wearing over 50 pounds) to do just 10 minutes on the stair climber, drop the vest down to 50 pounds and head over to a treadmill to finish up your 30 minutes with a fast walk. (I'm assuming that if your gym has a stair climber, it'll have a treadmill.) Or you could just go outside and walk quickly to get to your 30 minutes.

4. After you finish your Pre-Fatigue section, do any Mission workout. Now, doing pull-ups, push-ups, and kettle-bell movements with 50 pounds strapped to your back is going to very tough for most people. The rule here is that you need to do at least 3 good pull-ups and/or 5 push-ups, so you'll either have to take the vest off for this part or reduce the weight. You won't get much out of doing 1 pull-up or 3 push-ups. I highly recommend that you don't ever do the Mission section with any more than 50 pounds. In fact, unless you're a firefighter, you never need to go over 50 pounds for anything. I use 40 pounds as my standard vest weight; 25 pounds would be about right for most people to start with. I use 40 pounds because many years ago when I was in the infantry, an old gunnery sergeant told me to never let my pack go over 40 pounds. That number has been stuck in my head for almost 30 years. I still think it's a good rule.

Completing the rest of your Mission workout will be very tough with the extra weight, and all your reps will probably at least be about half of what you normally do. No biggie. Just go more slowly as you move around to prevent injury. You may think I'm being too cautious here, but I've busted my butt more than once wearing a full pack and/or a weighted vest. It's a whole different thing than just falling down without one. Your focus here is to train your body to handle the burden of extra weight you have to carry for your job, not to hit rep goals. Again, always train smart.

5. Finish this workout by doing your normal cool-down without the vest.

B. Outdoor Combo Workout

I put this session (and many variations like it) together to simulate a real-life working scenario. While it's geared toward firefighting movements, it's a great workout for anyone—a real nut buster if you push yourself. To really do this right you'll need some kettlebells and a length of rope (25 feet of 1-inch rope is about right). As I've said many times before, a set of kettlebells and a weighted vest are probably the best workout gear you could ever buy. They're almost like having a full-service gym that you can take anywhere. The amount of good PT you can get with these very simple pieces of gear is amazing. Nothing is more portable, effective, or more worth the money than those two items. If you don't have any kettlebells, you can use dumbbells or ammo cans for the Pre-Fatigue part, and a sea bag with some weight in it for the rope part. I like to use my 62-pound kettlebell for this, but you could use a sandbag or a small log—anything that's about 50–75 pounds that will drag across the ground without getting hung up.

1. Start with your normal warm-up without the vest.

2. Put on the vest and put your rope about 20–25 yards (you can go further if you'd like) away from your starting spot. Pick up your kettlebells, and jog or walk quickly to the rope. Once you get there, drop the kettlebells for a couple of seconds to catch your breath. Then do any kettlebell movement. Again, drop the kettlebells for a couple of seconds to catch your breath or, if you're a real hard ass, just take off for the other end without dropping them (going back to your starting point). Once there, as before, do one set of any kettlebell movement. Keep repeating this rotation until your 30 minutes are up. What I like to do is alternate a kettlebell movement on one end with a set of push-ups/pull-ups on the other. If you have a place to do pull-ups, obviously do those at that end. Keep moving back and forth non-stop. This will become true Pre-Fatigue in short order; stop and catch your breath only when you need to. Bring a water bottle and drink water throughout your workout.

3. After 30 minutes of that torture, grab your rope and tie off the two kettlebells (or whatever you brought for this) together. Jog out to the end of the rope, kneel down, and then drag the weight toward you. This simulates dragging in gear or a firehose. Get up and jog out to the end of the rope. Repeat this at least 3 times out and 3 times back as fast as you can. In between each lap, do a set of free squats. Next, put the rope behind you and run, dragging the weight. Jog up to the end of your course and come back 3 times; in between, do a set of mountain climbers.

4. Lastly, throw your rope over a low-hanging tree branch, jungle gym, or pull-up bar. Drop to your butt and hand over hand pull the weight up to the top. Lower them slowly. Do this 3 times with as little rest as you need between sets. Now take off your vest and do one 50-rep set of each of the 7 ab movements without stopping. All this should take you about 20 minutes if you kick it.

5. Trying not to collapse, catch your breath, get a drink of water, and do your cool-down.

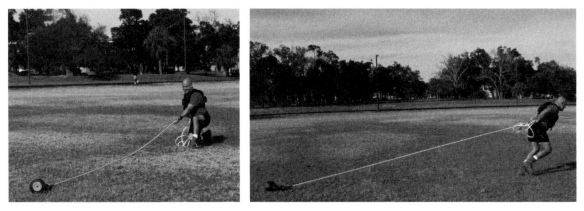

Part 3 of the Outdoor Combo Workout requires you to both reel your weight in and drag it behind you.

C. Forced March

For this hump (fast hike), you can wear a weighted vest or backpack. I prefer to wear a pack with about 40 pounds of weight. The vest is better for everything else, but I feel a pack is better for a hump. It just feels more natural to have all the weight on your back rather than straight down on your shoulders. I've done 20-plus-mile humps with a pack and at least 10 miles with a vest, so I'm speaking from experience. If you're regular infantry, I'm sure you don't need to practice this, but if you want to condition yourself for backpacking, it only makes sense that you use a pack as it more closely simulates your actual need. Either way, do your warm-up and then, with the vest/pack on, hike for at least an hour, up and down hills, through the woods, on the beach—whatever you can do to make it varied and tougher. You can do some short jogs at different points to vary the intensity. This is more of a toughening workout than anything else. This toughens your legs, back, and your shoulders where the weight rests like nothing else. If you're a real hard ass, push it out to 5, 10, or even more miles. It's a good workout but it takes some time, and you need to build up to it.

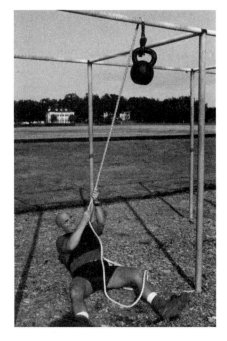

SCHEDULES

Here's an example of how a month's worth of EPRS may look. Of course, you can use these, but don't be tied down to a certain workout, to be done on a certain day. This is just an example based on 5 sessions a week (5 hours a week) with 2 days off.

Week 1

Monday	**SAT** > Pre-Fatigue—Track workout, Mission 1	
Tuesday	**Support** > Mountain bike ride (1 hour)	
Wednesday	**Off** (active rest—wash car)	
Thursday	**SAT** > Pre-Fatigue—Vest workout 1, Mission 2	
Friday	**Support** > MMA class	
Saturday	**Off** (active rest—golf)	
Sunday	**SAT** > Pre-Fatigue—Elliptical trainer, Mission 3	

Week 2

Monday	**SAT** > Pre-Fatigue—Treadmill, Mission 4	
Tuesday	**Support** > Lap swim (1 hour)	
Wednesday	**Off** (active rest—shoot baskets at the park)	
Thursday	**SAT** > Combo	
Friday	**Support** > Vest workout 2	
Saturday	**Support** > Beach volleyball (2–3 hours)	
Sunday	**Off** (active rest—mow lawn)	

Week 3

Monday	**SAT** > Pre-Fatigue—3-mile run, Mission 5
Tuesday	**Support** > Vest workout 3
Wednesday	**Off** (active rest—softball)
Thursday	**SAT** > Pre-Fatigue—stairwell with vest, Mission 6
Friday	**Support** > Boxing workout (1 hour)
Saturday	**Support** > Hike
Sunday	**Off** (active rest—beach)

Week 4

Monday	**SAT** > Pre-Fatigue—3-mile run on treadmill, Mission 7
Tuesday	**Support** > 5-mile jog (1 hour)
Wednesday	**Off** (active rest—long walk with dog)
Thursday	**SAT** > Pre-Fatigue—Rowing machine, Mission 1
Friday	**Support** > Yoga class (don't laugh till you try it)
Saturday	**Support** > Early a.m. bike ride (2 hours)
Sunday	**Off** > (active rest—fishing)

As you'll notice, I created as many different workouts as I could over the course of the month (in fact, these are much more varied than what I normally do). This was just to show you that you can be extremely flexible with different workouts and still stay within the guidelines of the system. If you do that and push yourself in the right places, at the right times, you'll get in some serious shape. It's important to note that while this seems like a lot of exercise, it never needs to be more than 5 hours a week. All the support workouts listed (like bike riding, hiking, and playing sports) are scheduled for at least a one-hour timeline. That's the minimum, but of course you can go much longer if you like and have the time (like I listed in some cases). I also listed the active rest I did on the "off" days. I plan things like washing the car and mowing the lawn on those days so I stay active and get all my "chores" done during the week. That way my weekends are free to goof off.

BASIC WARM-UP ROUTINE

This warm-up routine last approximately 5 minutes. For all of these moves, start by standing with your feet shoulder-width apart, unless noted otherwise.

Neck Rotations

Stand with your hands on your hips and slowly rotate your neck 5 times in each direction.

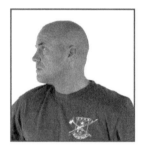
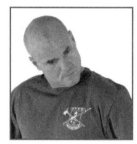

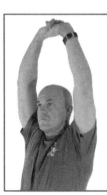

Overhead Stretch

Raise your arms overhead and stretch upward for a count of 5.

Chest Stretch

Clasp your hands together behind your back and slowly raise them to stretch your chest. Hold for a count of 5.

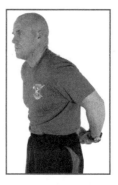

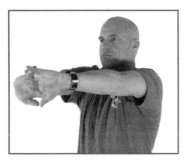

Back Stretch

Clasp your hands together in front of your body and raise them to chest level. Reach your arms forward to stretch your back. Hold for a count of 5.

High Elbow Stretch

Take one elbow up to the ceiling and next to your head. Slowly press down on your elbow with your other hand. Hold for a count of 5 with each arm.

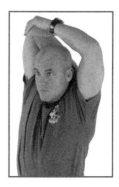

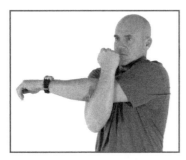

Low Elbow Stretch

Take one arm across your chest, hook your other arm under it, and pull your arm in toward your body. Hold for a count of 5 with each arm.

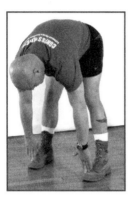

Hamstring Stretch

Fold forward, reaching toward your toes with your hands for a count of 5.

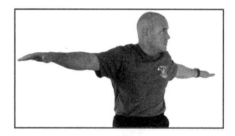

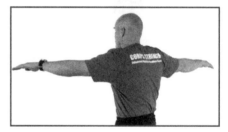

Side Twists

Extend your arms out to your sides and rotate your body to one side and then the other, twisting at the waist. One full rotation of your body (all the way to the left and the right) counts as one rep.

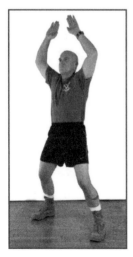

Side Straddle Hops (aka Jumping Jacks)

Stand with your feet together and your hands at your sides. With a jumping motion spread your legs and extend your arms over your head in an arc. Return to the starting position to complete one rep out of 5.

Arm Circles

Hold your arms in front of your body at shoulder height. Make large arm circles forward and backward. Do 5 circles in each direction.

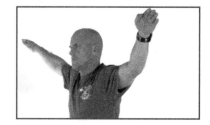

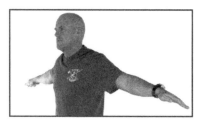

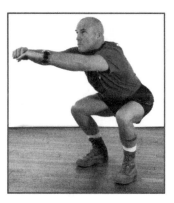

Free Squats

Perform 5 free squats (see page 95).

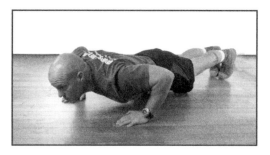

Push-Ups

Perform 5 regular push-ups (see page 85).

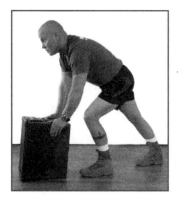

Achilles Stretch

Lean forward against any solid object (tree, car, wall, etc.) and take one leg forward and the other back. Bend your front leg until you feel the stretch in the back of your back leg. Hold for a count of 5, then switch legs.

BASIC COOL-DOWN ROUTINE

This cool-down routine last approximately 5 minutes.

Neck Rotations

Stand with your hands on your hips, feet shoulder-width apart, and slowly rotate your neck 5 times in each direction.

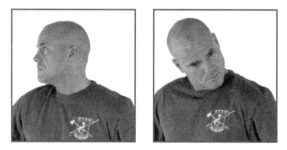

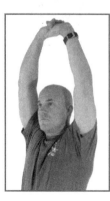

Overhead Stretch

Stand with your feet shoulder-width apart. Raise your arms overhead and stretch upward for a count of 10.

Chest Stretch

Stand with your feet shoulder-width apart. Clasp your hands together behind your back and slowly raise them to stretch your chest. Hold for a count of 10.

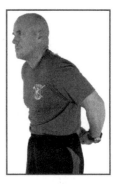

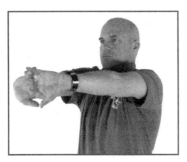

Back Stretch

Stand with your feet shoulder-width apart. Clasp your hands together in front of your body and raise them to chest level. Reach your arms forward to stretch your back. Hold for a count of 10.

High Elbow Stretch

Take one elbow up to the ceiling and next to your head. Slowly press down on your elbow with your other hand. Hold for a count of 5 with each arm.

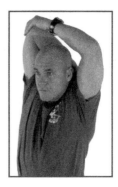

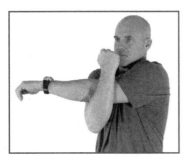

Low Elbow Stretch

Take one arm across your chest, hook your other arm under it, and pull your arm in toward your body. Hold for a count of 5 with each arm.

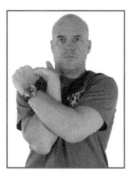

Wrist Stretch

Stand with your feet shoulder-width apart. Holding one elbow close to the front of your body, reach up with the opposite hand and grasp your hand at the fingertips. Slowly pull down on the fingers (press them backwards) to stretch the wrist. Hold each stretch for a count of 10.

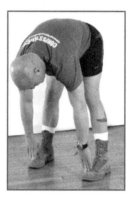

Hamstring Stretch

Stand with your feet shoulder-width apart. Fold forward, reaching toward your toes with your hands for a count of 10.

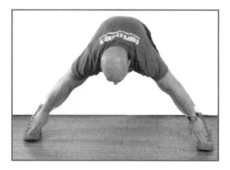

Wide Hamstring Stretch

This is the hamstring stretch with a slightly wider stance. Hold for a count of 10.

Very Wide Hamstring Stretch

This is the hamstring stretch with your widest stance. Hold for a count of 10.

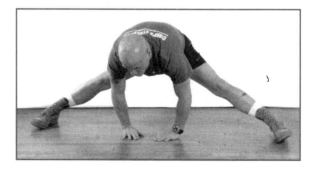

Seated Wide Stretch

Sit on the deck with your legs spread wide apart. Stretch by reaching forward on each leg and toward the center. Hold each position for a count of 10.

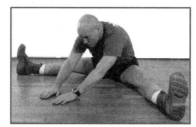 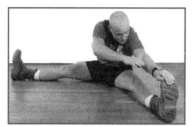

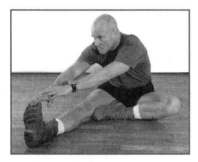

Modified Hurdler Stretch

Sit on the deck with your legs stretched out in front of you. Bring one leg in and reach toward the toe of the extended leg. Hold for a count of 10, then switch legs.

Seated Toe Touch

Sit on the deck with your legs stretched out in front of you. Reach for your toes and hold for a count of 10.

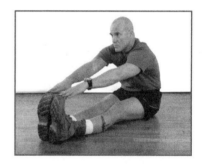

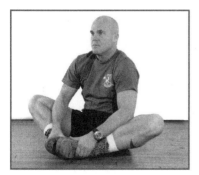

Indian Stretch

Sit with the soles of your feet together in front of your body. Grasp your toes and stretch your inner thighs by slowly pushing down on the insides of your knees. Hold for a count of 10. For an extra stretch, you can also slowly pull your head down toward your feet.

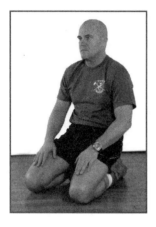

Seated Stretch

Sit with your feet folded under you and slowly lean back to stretch. Hold for a count of 10.

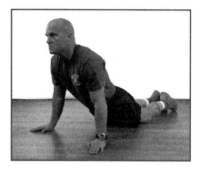

Cobra Stretch

Lie on your stomach with your hands beneath your shoulders. Keeping your elbows in, press yourself up until your chest is off the floor. Look upward to stretch your abdominals. Hold for a count of 10.

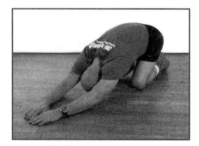

Cat Stretch

From the Cobra Stretch, press your hips back toward your heels and keep your arms extended forward. Hold for a count of 10.

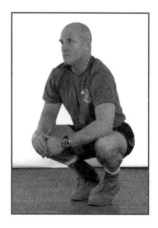

Squat Stretch

From the Cat Stretch, sit back into a squat position to stretch your ankles. Hold for a count of 10.

Alternating Hamstring Stretch

Stand and cross your left foot over your right. Fold over and slowly stretch the hamstrings of the back leg by reaching for your toes. Hold for a count of 10, then switch legs.

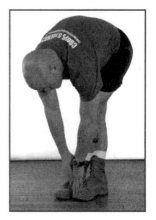

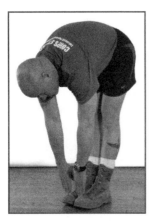

Toe Touch

Place both feet together and fold over to reach for your toes. Hold for a count of 10. Keeping your feet together makes it tougher.

Achilles Stretch

Lean forward against any solid object (tree, car, wall, etc.) and take one leg forward and the other back. Bend your front leg until you feel the stretch in the back of your back leg. Hold for a count of 10, then switch legs.

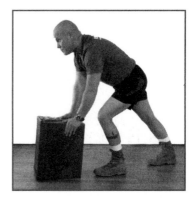

Bar Stretch (optional)

If you have a bench, bar, truck tailgate, etc., put one leg up and lean forward. Reach toward your toes to stretch your hamstrings. Hold for a count of 10, then switch legs.

INDEX

ACKNOWLEDGMENTS

At first glance the publication of a book seems pretty straightforward. That's not the reality. Lots of hard-working, talented people are needed to make this happen, and I've found that being the author may be the easiest part. I first have to thank my Marine, firefighter, and police officer friends (especially my fellow Marine buddies who endured some painful experimental workouts over the years), whose input and real-world experience helped me fine-tune my exercise system; their sweat, motivation, and support were greatly appreciated. A special thanks goes to Lori Tubbs, whose guidance on nutrition made it obvious to me just how much I have to learn on this subject. Thanks also to Gulf Beach Fitness and Omni Health and Fitness in Pensacola for the use of their gyms for all of the indoor pictures you see in the book; both are great places to PT. A big thank you must be given to my publisher Ulysses Press, not just for all their hard work in getting our book published, but for taking a chance on this hard-headed old Jarhead. Thanks, Keith, Claire, Lily, and Karma, for all your help and patience. Lastly I have to thank my wife Beverly, who has listened to a nonstop running monologue (including a fair amount of whining and complaining) about this idea for over a year. Despite hearing it dozens of times over, she never tired or waivered in her support for me. I love you, Bev.

ABOUT THE AUTHOR

Paul Roarke Jr. was born in Troy, New York, and enlisted in the United States Marine Corps in 1981. Over the next 28 years, Paul served around the world and in the United States as an active-duty Marine, including combat operations in Desert Storm, Kosovo, and Iraq. Retiring in 2009 as a Master Gunnery Sergeant, Paul published this book based on his long experience in physical-readiness training. Paul is presently employed as a physical training and leadership instructor at the Naval International Training Center in Pensacola, Florida, where he lives with his wife and two sons.